T0228996

Hemoglobin-based Oxygen Carriers (HBOCs): The Future in Resuscitation?

Guest Editor

LENA M. NAPOLITANO, MD

CRITICAL CARE CLINICS

www.criticalcare.theclinics.com

Consulting Editors
RICHARD W. CARLSON, MD, PhD
MICHAEL A. GEHEB, MD

April 2009 • Volume 25 • Number 2

SAUNDERS an imprint of ELSEVIER, Inc.

W.B. SAUNDERS COMPANY
A Division of Elsevier Inc.

Elsevier Inc. • 1600 John F. Kennedy Blvd., • Suite 1800 • Philadelphia, Pennsylvania 19103-2899

http://www.theclinics.com

CRITICAL CARE CLINICS Volume 25, Number 2
April 2009 ISSN 0749-0704, ISBN-13: 978-1-4377-0462-4, ISBN-10: 1-4377-0462-X

Editor: Patrick Manley
Developmental Editor: Donald Mumford

Critical Care Clinics (ISSN: 0749-0704) is published quarterly by Elsevier Inc., 360 Park Avenue South, New York, NY 10010-1710. Months of issue are January, April, July, and October. Business and Editorial Offices: 1600 John F. Kennedy Blvd., Suite 1800, Philadelphia, PA 19103-2899. Customer Service Office: 6277 Sea Harbor Drive, Orlando, FL 32887-4800. Periodicals postage paid at New York, NY and additional mailing offices. Subscription prices are $222.00 per year for US individuals, $366.00 per year for US institution, $111.00 per year for US students and residents, $274.00 per year for Canadian individuals, $454.00 per year for Canadian institutions, $320.00 per year for international individuals, $454.00 per year for international institutions and $161.00 per year for Canadian and foreign students/residents. To receive student/resident rate, orders must be accompanied by name of affiliated institution, date of term, and the *signature* of program/residency coordinator on institution letterhead. Orders will be billed at individual rate until proof of status is received. Foreign air speed delivery is included in all *Clinics* subscription prices. All prices are subject to change without notice. POSTMASTER: Send address changes to *Critical Care Clinics*, Elsevier Periodicals Customer Service, 11830 Westline Industrial Drive, St. Louis, MO 63146. **Customer Service: 1-800-654-2452 (US). From outside of the US, call 1-314-453-7041. Fax: 1-314-453-5170. E-mail: journalscustomerservice-usa@elsevier.com (for print support) or journalsonlinesupport-usa@elsevier.com (for online support).**

Reprints. For copies of 100 or more of articles in this publication, please contact the Commercial Reprints Department, Elsevier Inc., 360 Park Avenue South, New York, NY 10010-1710. Tel.: 212-633-3812; Fax: 212-462-1935; E-mail: reprints@elsevier.com.

Critical Care Clinics is also published in Spanish by Editorial Inter-Medica, Junin 917, 1er A, 1113, Buenos Aires, Argentina.

Critical Care Clinics is covered in *MEDLINE/PubMed (Index Medicus), EMBASE/Excerpta Medica, Current Concepts/Clinical Medicine, ISI/BIOMED, and Chemical Abstracts.*

Printed and bound by CPI Group (UK) Ltd, Croydon, CR0 4YY

Transferred to Digital Print 2011

Contributors

CONSULTING EDITORS

RICHARD W. CARLSON, MD, PhD
Chairman, Department of Internal Medicine, Marcopia Medical Center; and Professor, Department of Medicine, Mayo Graduate School of Medicine, Phoenix, Arizona

MICHAEL A. GEHEB, MD
Professor, Department of Medicine, and Vice President, Clinical Programs, Oregon Health & Sciences University, Portland, Oregon

GUEST EDITOR

LENA M. NAPOLITANO, MD, FACS, FCCP, FCCM
Director, Surgical Critical Care Trauma, University of Michigan; and Professor of Surgery, Division Chief, Acute Care Surgery, Associate Chair, Division of Acute Care Surgery, Department of Surgery, University of Michigan, Ann Arbor, Michigan

AUTHORS

T.M.S. CHANG, OC, MD, CM, PhD, FRCPC, FRS(C)
Professor and Director, Artificial Cells and Organs Research Center, Faculty of Medicine, McGill University, Montreal, Quebec, Canada

CLAUDIA S. COHN, MD, PhD
House Officer IV, Department of Pathology, New York Presbyterian Hospital/Weill-Cornell, New York, New York

JACQUES CRETEUR, MD, PhD
Associate Professor, Department of Intensive Care, Erasme Hospital, Université libre de Bruxelles, Brussels, Belgium

MELISSA M. CUSHING, MD
Assistant Professor, Department of Pathology, Weill Cornell Medical College, New York, New York

LUC DOUAY, MD, PhD
Professor, UMR-S 938, Université Pierre et Marie Curie, Paris, France

ALEXANDER L. EASTMAN, MD
Fellow in Surgical Critical Care, Department of Surgery, Division of Burn, Trauma and Critical Care, University of Texas Southwestern Medical Center, Dallas, Texas

CLARA FRONTICELLI, PhD
Professor, Department of Anesthesiology and Critical Care Medicine, The Johns Hopkins University School of Medicine, Baltimore, Maryland

A. GERSON GREENBURG, MD, PhD
Vice President, Medical Affairs, Biopure Corporation, Cambridge, Massachusetts;
Professor of Surgery, Emeritus, Brown

LAWRENCE TIM GOODNOUGH, MD
Professor of Pathology and Medicine, Department of Pathology, Stanford University
Medical Center, Stanford, California

JEFFREY L. JOHNSON, MD
Department of Surgery, Denver Health Medical Center, University of Colorado Health
Sciences Center, Denver, Colorado

RAYMOND C. KOEHLER, PhD
Professor, Department of Anesthesiology and Critical Care Medicine, The Johns Hopkins
University School of Medicine, Baltimore, Maryland

HÉLÈNE LAPILLONNE, MD, PhD
Service d'Hématologie biologique, AP-HP, Hôpital d'enfants Armand Trousseau and
UPMC Univ. Paris 06, UMR_S938, Paris, France

JOSEPH P. MINEI, MD
Professor and Vice Chair, Department of Surgery, Division of Burn, Trauma and Critical
Care, University of Texas Southwestern Medical Center; and Surgeon-in-Chief, Parkland
Memorial Hospital, Dallas, Texas

ERNEST E. MOORE, MD
Chief, Department of Surgery, Denver Health Medical Center, University of Colorado
Health Sciences Center, Denver, Colorado

FREDERICK A. MOORE, MD
Department of Surgery, Methodist Hospital and Weill-Cornell University, Houston, Texas

HUNTER B. MOORE, BA
University of Vermont School of Medicine, Burlington, Vermont

LENA M. NAPOLITANO, MD, FACS, FCCP, FCCM
Director, Surgical Critical Care Trauma, University of Michigan; and Professor of Surgery,
Division Chief, Acute Care Surgery, Associate Chair, Division of Acute Care Surgery,
Department of Surgery, University of Michigan, Ann Arbor, Michigan

ARYEH SHANDER, MD
Chief, Department of Anesthesiology, Critical Care, and Hyperbaric Medicine,
Englewood Hospital and Medical Center, Englewood, New Jersey; Clinical Professor,
Departments of Anesthesiology, Medicine, and Surgery, Mount Sinai School of Medicine,
New York, New York

ALI G. TURHAN, MD, PhD
Division of Laboratory Hematology and Oncology, University of Poitiers, Poitiers, France

JEAN-LOUIS VINCENT, MD, PhD
Professor, Department of Intensive Care, Erasme Hospital, Université libre de Bruxelles,
Brussels, Belgium

Contents

Preface   **xi**

Lena M. Napolitano

Why an Alternative to Blood Transfusion?   **261**

Aryeh Shander and Lawrence Tim Goodnough

> Allogeneic blood transfusions have been associated with several risks and
> complications and with worse outcomes in a substantial number of patient
> populations and clinical scenarios. Allogeneic blood is costly and difficult
> to procure, transport, and store. Global and local shortages are imminent.
> Alternatives to transfusion provide many advantages, and their use is likely
> to improve outcomes as safer and more effective agents are developed.

Hemoglobin-based Oxygen Carriers: First, Second or Third Generation?
Human or Bovine? Where are we Now?   **279**

Lena M. Napolitano

> This article discusses current efforts to develop hemoglobin-based
> oxygen carriers as blood substitutes in light of the worldwide shortage of
> safe and viable allogeneic donor blood. There are now viable approaches
> to modify the intrinsic biologic properties of hemoglobin to produce
> improved hemoglobin-based oxygen carriers. Polymerized hemoglobin
> preparations have proved most successful in clinical trials due to their
> improved side effect profile. The goal is to evaluate blood substitutes
> with enhanced intravascular retention, reduced osmotic activity, and
> attenuated hemodynamic derangements such as vasoconstriction.
> Although not without substantial morbidity and mortality, the current safety
> of allogeneic blood transfusion demands that comparative studies show
> minimal adverse effects as well as efficacy and potential for novel
> applications.

Comparison of Hemoglobin-based Oxygen Carriers to Stored Human
Red Blood Cells   **303**

Alexander L. Eastman and Joseph P. Minei

> Since the inception of allogeneic blood transfusion, the search for an
> alternative to the use of stored packed red blood cells has been underway.
> Over the last 10 years, modified hemoglobin solutions in the form of hemo-
> globin-based oxygen carriers (HBOCs) have made significant strides
> toward becoming clinically available and useful. Although HBOCs are
> not yet ready for regular use in the clinical arena, this may change in the
> near future as HBOC products continue to improve and as the elucidation
> of the mechanisms of any adverse effects becomes clearer. In the mean
> time, we must further the development of alternative strategies for the
> "hemoglobin bridge" so desperately needed by many critically ill patients.

Potential Uses of Hemoglobin-based Oxygen Carriers in Critical Care Medicine 311

Jacques Creteur and Jean-Louis Vincent

Hemoglobin-based oxygen carriers (HBOCs) were initially developed to provide an alternative to blood transfusion. With the realization that hemoglobin solutions not only are red blood cell substitutes but also have a number of additional properties, including hemodynamic effects related to their oncotic and nitric oxide–scavenging effects, the broader concept of "hemoglobin therapeutics" was born. Promising effects on oxygen transport and the microcirculation need to be confirmed, and the results of studies with newer, second-generation HBOCs are eagerly awaited. In the meantime, possible adverse effects need to be carefully evaluated before HBOCs can be widely used in the ICU, emergency room, or prehospital setting.

The USA Multicenter Prehospital Hemoglobin-based Oxygen Carriers Resuscitation Trial: Scientific Rationale, Study Design, and Results 325

Ernest E. Moore, Jeffrey L. Johnson, Fredrick A. Moore, and Hunter B. Moore

Human polymerized hemoglobin (PolyHeme) is a universally compatible oxygen carrier developed for use when red blood cells are unavailable and oxygen-carrying replacement is needed to treat life-threatening anemia. This multicenter phase III trial assessed survival of patients resuscitated with a hemoglobin-based oxygen carrier starting at the scene of injury. Patients resuscitated with PolyHeme had outcomes comparable to those receiving the standard of care including rapid access to stored red blood cells. Although there were more adverse events in the PolyHeme group compared with control patients receiving blood, the observed safety profile is acceptable for the intended population. The benefit-to-risk ratio of PolyHeme is favorable when blood is needed but is not available or an option.

Design of Recombinant Hemoglobins for Use in Transfusion Fluids 357

Clara Fronticelli and Raymond C. Koehler

Molecular biology has been applied to the development of hemoglobin-based oxygen carrier (HBOC) proteins that can be expressed in bacteria or yeast. The transformation of the hemoglobin molecule into an HBOC requires a variety of modifications for rendering the acellular molecule of hemoglobin physiologically acceptable when transfused in circulation. Hemoglobins with different oxygen affinities can be obtained by introducing mutations at the heme pocket, the site of oxygen binding, or by introducing surface mutations that stabilize the hemoglobin molecule in the low-oxygen-affinity state. Modification of the size of the heme pocket is also used to hinder nitric oxide depletion and associated vasoconstriction. Introduction of cysteine residues on the hemoglobin surface allows formation of intermolecular bonds and formation of polymeric HBOCs. These polymers of recombinant hemoglobin have the characteristics of molecular size, molecular stability, and oxygen delivery to hypoxic tissue suitable for an HBOC.

Nanobiotechnology for Hemoglobin-based Blood Substitutes   373

T.M.S. Chang

Nanobiotechnology is the assembling of biological molecules into nanodimension complexes. This has been used for the preparation of polyhemoglobin formed by the assembling of hemoglobin molecules into a soluble nanodimension complex. New generations of this approach include the nanobiotechnological assembly of hemoglobin, catalase, and superoxide dismutase into a soluble nanodimension complex. This acts as an oxygen carrier and an antioxidant for those conditions with potential for ischemiareperfusion injuries. Another recent novel approach is the assembling of hemoglobin and fibrinogen into a soluble nanodimension polyhemoglobin-fibrinogen complex that acts as an oxygen carrier with platelet-like activity. This is potentially useful in cases of extensive blood loss requiring massive replacement using blood substitutes, resulting in the need for the replacement of platelets and clotting factors. A further step is the preparation of nanodimension artificial red blood cells that contain hemoglobin and all the enzymes present in red blood cells.

Stem Cells—A Source of Adult Red Blood Cells for Transfusion Purposes: Present and Future   383

Luc Douay, Hélène Lapillonne, and Ali G. Turhan

We have sufficient knowledge of the biology of hematopoietic stem cells to hope that we might generate human red blood cells in the laboratory. It may soon be possible to produce enough to transfuse "cultured" red blood cells to manufacture human red blood cells from hematopoietic stem cells for transfusion purposes. This article describes progress and the challenges that remain in the search for in vitro generated red blood cells that can be efficiently manufactured in high volumes and given to any recipient.

Oxygen Therapeutics: Perfluorocarbons and Blood Substitute Safety   399

Claudia S. Cohn and Melissa M. Cushing

Current demands over the blood supply in developed and developing nations will compound over time. Red cell substitutes have a promising value proposition for transfusion services, because they hold the promise of increasing the availability of blood products and removing donor and contamination safety risks. In this article, the authors note that existing products suffer from critical shortcomings such as vasoactivity; they also point out that substitutes not based on human blood introduce potentially more complex safety hurdles. The authors discuss the attributes of an ideal blood substitute, and the mechanism and current status of perfluorocarbons; they also review the shortcomings of all oxygen therapeutic products in development today.

The Ideal Blood Substitute   **415**

A. Gerson Greenberg

There is an ongoing need for a red cell substitute, an oxygen-carrying solution to use primarily as a bridge until red cells are available. The replacement of oxygen-carrying capacity has driven the field of research, primarily with the development of hemoglobin-based oxygen carriers, but they are less than ideal. The formulation of a complete substitute for blood, if it can be realized, must take into account all the cellular and molecular components of the immune and coagulation systems.

Index   **425**

FORTHCOMING ISSUES

July 2009
Sedation and Analgesia in Critically Ill Patients
Pratik Pandharipande, MD,
and E. Wesley Ely, MD,
Guest Editors

October 2009
Sepsis
Phillip Dellinger, MD,
Guest Editor

January 2010
Intensive Care of the Cancer Patient
Stephen M. Pastores, MD,
and Neil Halpern, MD,
Guest Editors

RECENT ISSUES

January 2009
Historical Aspects of Critical Illness and Critical Care Medicine
Anand Kumar, MD,
and Joseph Parrillo, MD,
Guest Editors

October 2008
Psychiatric Aspects of Critical Care Medicine
Jose R. Maldonado, MD,
Guest Editor

July 2008
Sleep in the ICU
Nancy A. Collup, MD,
Guest Editor

RELATED INTEREST

Emergency Medicine Clinics of North America Volume 27, Issue 1, February 2009
Neurologic Emergencies
Robert Silbergleit, MD, and Romergryko Geocadin, MD, *Guest Editors*

THE CLINICS ARE NOW AVAILABLE ONLINE!
Access your subscription at:
www.theclinics.com

Preface

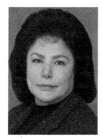

Lena M. Napolitano, MD, FACS, FCCP, FCCM
Guest Editor

The need for an alternative to allogeneic red blood cells for transfusion has been recognized for more than a century. The most serious motivation for the development of a blood substitute is the worldwide shortage of safe and viable allogeneic donor blood.

More than 14 million units of allogeneic blood are transfused in the United States annually. The number of red blood cell units transfused in 2006 was 14,650,000 units, reflecting a 40% increase in red blood cell transfusions compared with 1994 (10.5 million units) and a 3.3% increase in transfusion activity from 2004. Autologous blood collection declined significantly during this same period by 26.9% to 335,000 units. A significant portion of these transfusions are administered to critically ill patients in the intensive care unit (ICU). Multiple studies have confirmed that approximately 45% of critically ill patients are transfused with an average of four to five units of red blood cells during their ICU stay.

Blood acquisition costs have more than doubled in the past few years and are likely to continue to increase as the blood supply struggles to meet the increasing demand. In response to a sharply increasing demand for red blood cells for transfusion, research into alternatives to red blood cell transfusion is necessary. The development of a blood substitute, an intravenous solution that does not require refrigeration or cross-matching, has a long shelf life, and is associated with reduced risk of iatrogenic infection, would provide a potentially lifesaving option for surgical and trauma patients with hemorrhagic shock, especially in settings in which blood is not available. The blood substitutes that have reached advanced clinical trials today are red blood cell substitutes derived from hemoglobin, specifically polymerized hemoglobin-based oxygen carrier (HBOC) solutions.

In this issue of the *Critical Care Clinics of North America*, the evidence regarding HBOCs, their efficacy and potential toxicities, results of clinical trials, and other potential blood substitutes in active development is reviewed. The first section addresses the issue of why an alternative to blood transfusion is needed. Next, we review the differences in the earlier and more recent HBOCs, their hemoglobin sources (human or bovine), results of HBOC clinical trials done to date, recombinant hemoglobin update, cellular HBOCs, and adverse effects of HBOCs. Additional information comparing HBOCs with stored human red blood cells is next. Most importantly,

Crit Care Clin 25 (2009) xi–xii
doi:10.1016/j.ccc.2009.02.002
0749-0704/09/$ – see front matter

potential uses of HBOCs in critical care are reviewed, and the results of the recent US multicenter prehospital trauma trial are carefully detailed by the lead investigators. Important ongoing research regarding recombinant hemoglobins, nanobiotechnology for HBOCs, stem cells as a source of adult red blood cells, and perfluorocarbons is reviewed in detail. A section on safety, adverse events, and toxicities related to HBOCs is extremely important. The final section provides perspectives on the "ideal blood substitute."

The development of a safe and effective blood substitute is of great importance to critical care medicine in civilian and military medicine. The full scope of the science and technology of HBOCs and other blood substitutes has grown to such an extent that no single issue of the *Clinics* can fully address the topic, but we are hopeful that this issue acts as a base for further reading and research.

I would like to thank the authors for generously contributing their time and expertise in the preparation of this issue. I would also like to acknowledge Dr. Richard Carlson and the Elsevier editorial staff for their tireless support and assistance in bringing this issue to completion. I sincerely hope that this issue serves as a timely and current reference to assist critical care practitioners in the pursuit of knowledge in this field.

Lena M. Napolitano, MD, FACS, FCCP, FCCM
Department of Surgery
University of Michigan Medical Center
1500 East Medical Center Drive
1C421 University Hospital, Box 0033
Ann Arbor, MI 48109–0033, USA

E-mail address:
lenan@umich.edu

Why an Alternative to Blood Transfusion?

Aryeh Shander, MD[a,b,*], Lawrence Tim Goodnough, MD[c]

KEYWORDS

- Transfusion • Risk • Cost • Outcome
- Allogeneic • Complication

Apart from the Hippocratic Oath, many fail to appreciate the deep marks left by Hippocrates on medicine. For one, he is credited with applying humorism to medicine and putting forth the idea that imbalances among the humors were responsible for human diseases. Being one of the four humors, blood has mesmerized people throughout history. This preoccupation has occasionally surfaced through colorful and horrifying stories of primitive attempts at transferring blood among and between humans and animals. In many accounts, such as the renowned story of the ailing Pope Innocent VIII receiving blood from young boys to rejuvenate, it is hard to discern fact from fiction. Yet, there is no doubt that blood has always been believed to be associated with life and vitality and key to curing numerous ailments.

Old habits die hard. For many physicians, ordering allogeneic blood transfusions is a matter of little hesitation. The belief that blood transfusion is a quick and easy way to boost a patient's condition and accelerate recovery is held by many. Faced with more and more evidence on the lack of safety and efficacy of blood transfusions, however, it is becoming increasingly clear that such beliefs are largely unsubstantiated and tainted with myths. For these reasons, allogeneic transfusions should be minimized. Moreover, there are situations in which blood transfusions are simply not available or acceptable to patients. In even a greater number of cases, although allogeneic blood may be available with little objection from patients, giving transfusions may

Aryeh Shander has been or is currently a paid consultant for Biopure, Bayer, Hemo Concepts, NovoNordisk, OrthoBiotech, and ZymoGenetics; has received grants/research support from Abbott, AstraZeneca, OrthoBiotech, and ZymoGenetics; and has received speaking honorariums from Baxter, Bayer, Pfizer, Hemo Concepts, NovoNordisk, OrthoBiotech, and ZymoGenetics. Lawrence Tim Goodnough has been or is a paid consultant for Amgen, OrthoBiotech, American regent, Watson Pharm, and Eli Lilly.

[a] Department of Anesthesiology, Critical Care and Hyperbaric Medicine, Englewood Hospital and Medical Center, 350 Engle Street, Englewood, NJ 07631, USA
[b] Departments of Anesthesiology, Medicine and Surgery, Mount Sinai School of Medicine, NY, USA
[c] Departments of Pathology and Medicine, Stanford University Medical Center, 300 Pasteur Drive, Room H-1402, MC 5626, Stanford, CA 94305, USA
* Corresponding author. Department of Anesthesiology, Critical Care and Hyperbaric Medicine, Englewood Hospital and Medical Center, 350 Engle Street, Englewood, NJ 07631, USA.
E-mail address: aryeh.shander@ehmc.com (A. Shander).

expose them to increased risks and bring about undesired outcomes. Therefore, alternatives to allogeneic blood should be sought. This article looks at the evidence for and against the use of allogeneic transfusions and discusses why alternatives to transfusion are needed.

PHYSIOLOGY OF OXYGEN TRANSPORT, ANEMIA, AND TRANSFUSION

For over a billion years, oxygen was little more than a toxic waste product of photosynthetic reactions. Some two billion years ago, as oxygen levels in the atmosphere began to rise, organisms developed the revolutionary capability to use oxygen as the ultimate electron acceptor. Aerobic metabolism provided a much more efficient way of releasing energy compared with fermentation and paved the way for the evolution of much more complicated, multicellular organisms.[1] As the size of multicellular organisms increased, simple diffusion could not keep up with oxygen demand, and ingenious mechanisms for transporting oxygen were developed. An indicator of the importance of such mechanisms (and their development early on in evolution) is the presence of various related hemoglobin (Hb) molecules in species ranging from plants to humans.[2]

Human Hb in adults consists of two alpha and two beta chains, each harboring an oxygen-binding heme group. Thus, each Hb molecule is capable of binding up to four oxygen molecules, which would amount to 1.39 mL of oxygen binding per gram of Hb at 37°C. The binding of oxygen to Hb is cooperative, and the affinity changes depending on the oxygen saturation status of the tetramer. The result is a sigmoid Hb oxygen dissociation curve with a steep slope in lower oxygen partial pressures (PO_2; range 20–40 mm Hg) usually seen in peripheral tissues, followed by a gradual turn into a plateau as PO_2 approaches the levels present in the alveolus (**Fig. 1**). The affinity for oxygen is further affected by other factors such as pH and

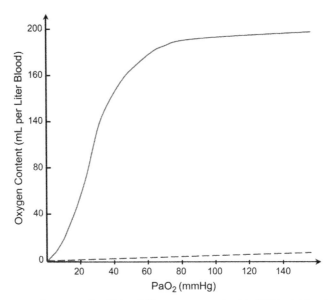

Fig. 1. Oxygen-carrying capacity of blood. The oxygen content in 1000 mL blood with 150 g/L Hb at various PaO_2 levels. Solid and dashed lines represent the Hb-bound and plasma-dissolved oxygen, respectively.

2,3-diphosphoglycerate; this is in contrast to oxygen being dissolved in a fluid (eg, plasma), which is a linear function of PO_2 according to Henry's law (see **Fig. 1**). Oxygen in blood is carried in Hb-bound and in plasma-dissolved forms, and thus the total oxygen content of arterial blood (CaO_2) is calculated as the sum of these two:

$$CaO_2 = \text{Total Hb-bound oxygen} + \text{Total plasma-dissolved oxygen} = ([Hb] \times SaO_2$$
$$\times \text{Hb oxygen binding capacity}) + (PaO_2 \times \text{plasma oxygen solubility}) \quad (1)$$

where CaO_2 is the actual oxygen content of arterial blood, *[Hb]* is the concentration of Hb in blood, SaO_2 is the arterial oxygen saturation of Hb, and PaO_2 is the arterial oxygen partial pressure.[3] At 37°C, Hb oxygen binding capacity is 1.39 mL/g and plasma oxygen solubility is 0.0031 mL/(dL·mm Hg).[4]

As evident from **Fig. 1**, within physiologic ranges of PaO_2, the amount of oxygen dissolved in plasma is negligible relative to Hb-bound oxygen and can be ignored. It should be pointed out, however, that under special circumstances (eg, treatment with hyperbaric oxygen or infusion of perfluorocarbons in the context of low Hb), plasma-dissolved oxygen can become a major source for supplying oxygen to the tissues.

Oxygen delivery to tissues (DO_2) is a product of blood oxygen content (calculated from Equation 1) and cardiac output (CO), which can be written in the following simplified equation under physiologic conditions:

$$DO_2 = \{[Hb] \times SaO_2 \times 1.39\} \times CO \quad (2)$$

Based on this equation, DO_2 appears to be directly related to [Hb] and one would deduce that any drop in [Hb] would result in reduced DO_2. Moreover, assuming that Hb is almost entirely saturated with oxygen, the easiest way to increase DO_2 appears to be to increase [Hb]. This notion has been the core physiologic justification behind giving blood transfusions to anemic patients.[5]

Such would be the case if we were considering a closed and static system of tubes and reservoirs. In reality, however, circulation is a dynamic system with far more complexity, and the relationship between [Hb] and DO_2 is anything but a direct linear one. Anemia is associated with physiologic adaptations that substantially diminish the effect of reduced [Hb] on DO_2. Studies in healthy individuals have shown that when isovolemia is maintained, an acute decrease in [Hb] to as low as 4 to 5 g/dL is well tolerated with no sign of tissue hypoxia. In these cases, circulatory response is characterized by decreased systemic vascular resistance, increased heart rate, and increased stroke volume.[6] Other changes observed in this setting include increased preload and decreased afterload due to reduced blood viscosity,[7] and inotropic sympathetic stimulation of heart.[8] All these changes result in increased COut at the level of the macrocirculation that, according to Equation 2, offsets the negative effect of reduced [Hb] on DO_2.

Furthermore, it should be remembered that normally in the microcirculation, where the blood cells pass through vessels with decreasing diameters, the de facto hematocrit becomes substantially lower than the laboratory-measured hematocrit due to more optimal alignment of red blood cells (RBCs) with the flow (the Fahraeus-Lindqvist effect).[9] This microcirculatory hematocrit stays essentially unchanged despite a significant decrease of hematocrit in the macrocirculation. Under physiologic conditions, the oxygen transported and delivered by blood (ie, DO_2) far exceeds the required oxygen actually consumed by the organs (oxygen consumption; $\dot{V}O_2$) by a factor of three to five, resulting in an oxygen extraction ratio of merely 20% to 30%. This large reserve capacity means that $\dot{V}O_2$ is largely unaffected by a drop in DO_2 (and [Hb]) until a critical low [Hb] is reached.[4,10] In addition, hemodilution is shown to be associated with microcirculatory changes and a shift of the Hb-oxygen dissociation curve to the right, resulting in higher oxygen extraction at peripheral tissues.[11,12] It has been suggested, however, that the response to anemia at the microvascular level is organ specific, and each organ may have a different tolerance to anemia.[13] Although the lowest [Hb] below which $\dot{V}O_2$ is compromised is an elusive value dependent on many factors, for all practical purposes, this critical [Hb] level is lower (significantly, in many cases) than the arbitrary [Hb] of 10 g/dL (hematocrit of 30%) suggested as the transfusion trigger by the outdated "10/30" rule.

On the other hand, other factors may adversely affect tolerance of low [Hb]. While reduced viscosity as a result of anemia is associated with increased COut, data from studies mostly done in animal models indicate that a minimum blood viscosity is required to maintain microvascular perfusion and functional capillary density. To this end, it has been suggested that blood viscosity may be more important than its oxygen-carrying capacity in determining the critical [Hb] and the lowest RBC concentration that can be tolerated.[14] Moreover, many agents used in anesthesia can blunt the adaptive circulatory mechanisms in response to anemia,[15] although it should be pointed out that reduced activity in an anesthetized patient also reduces oxygen demand. Finally, special cases, such as patients who have heart failure and coronary artery disease and elderly patients who may have reduced tolerance to anemia, may require more vigilance.[4,16,17] This notion, however, has not been supported in studies: better ischemic outcomes in elderly patients or patients who had active cardiac disease were not seen in transfused compared with nontransfused patients, even among those who had a nadir hematocrit below 21%.[18–21]

Studies looking into the effectiveness of blood transfusions in augmenting oxygenation parameters have had mixed results. A review of 18 studies indicated that although [Hb] invariably increased following transfusion in all studies, increased DO_2 was observed in 14 studies and increased $\dot{V}O_2$ (the parameter that really matters) was detected in just five studies.[22,23] A plausible explanation might be the lack of a real need for transfusion in most of the patients in these studies, because giving additional blood is not likely to increase a $\dot{V}O_2$ level that is already within the normal range.[22]

Therefore, the question of usefulness and efficacy of blood transfusions ultimately boils down to the issue of the transfusion indications. In anemic/bleeding patients who have been adequately managed to maintain isovolemia and to avoid/treat tachycardia (and in the absence of other probable causes), evidence of organ ischemia (eg, new ST-segment depression >0.1 mV or elevation >0.2 mV, new wall-motion abnormality), inadequate blood oxygen content (eg, mixed venous partial pressure of oxygen <32 mm Hg, mixed venous oxygen saturation <60%), or compromised oxygen consumption (more than 10% decrease in $\dot{V}O_2$, oxygen extraction ratio >40%) may indicate the need for blood transfusion, although definitive data to support the positive outcome of transfusion are not available.[22] A number of criteria based on [Hb] have also been suggested to guide transfusion;[24] however, it is evident from the evidence discussed here that physiologic triggers are more accurate indicators of an individual patient need for blood, as opposed to one-size-fits-all [Hb]-based triggers. It is hoped that further research on tolerance of anemia and indicators of ischemia will provide better indicators to guide transfusion decisions and to identify patients who are most likely to benefit from blood and the far greater number who do not need transfusion and are harmed by it.

RISKS OF TRANSFUSION

Despite being considered a mundane and commonplace practice, allogeneic blood transfusion is essentially a form of organ transplantation. The risks of transfusion have been long recognized, as evidenced by the bans on transfusion in England and France in the seventeenth and eighteenth centuries. Later on, as discovery of blood groups paved the way for successful transfusions, other complications such as transfusion-transmitted jaundice began to surface. Subsequently, donor screening procedures and tests were implemented, greatly improving the safety of blood.

Transfusion risks can be categorized into infectious and noninfectious risks. Noninfectious risks are furthered grouped into immunologic and nonimmunologic risks (**Table 1**).[25] As a result of continuously improved screening and testing, the blood supply today is safer than ever from infectious risks. Nonetheless, the risk is not yet zero (and it is unlikely to be zero any time soon) because many infections have windows during which they are not readily detectable by tests. Moreover, there is always the possibility of new, emerging infections lurking around that will not be tested for until their risk is recognized and adequate testing has been developed for them.[29] Currently,

Table 1	
Potential risks of transfusion	
Category	**Risks**
Infectious	Viral infections (hepatitis A, B, C, E, and G; HIV-1 and -2; HTLV-1 and -2; HHV-8; cytomegalovirus; Epstein-Barr virus; parvovirus B19)
	Bacterial (syphilis, tick-borne infections, contamination)
	Prion (Creutzfeldt-Jakob disease, new variant)
	Parasitic (malaria, babesiosis, Chagas' disease)
	Agents not yet discovered or screened for (emerging pathogens)
Noninfectious	
Immunologic	Multiple organ failure/dysfunction syndrome attributed to cytokine release
	Postoperative infection
	Transfusion-associated sepsis
	Increased risk of cancer recurrence
	Down-regulation of macrophage and T-cell function
	HLA alloimmunization
	Transfusion-associated graft-versus-host disease
	Hemolytic transfusion reactions (immunologic)
	Allergic and anaphylactic reactions
Nonimmunologic	Transfusion errors
	Febrile nonhemolytic transfusion reactions
	Posttransfusion purpura
	Hemolytic transfusion reactions (nonimmunologic)
	Risks of old blood (storage lesion, microcirculatory occlusion, lack of effectiveness)
	Circulatory overload
	Iron overload
	Hypotensive reactions
	Metabolic disturbances (citrate toxicity, hypocalcemia, hyperkalemia, acidosis, hyperammonemia)
	Hypothermia

Abbreviations: HHV, human herpesvirus; HTLV, human T-lymphotropic virus.
Data from Refs. [9,25–28]

infective agents for which donated blood is usually tested include hepatitis B (HBV), hepatitis C (HCV), HIV-1 and -2, human T-lymphotropic virus (HTLV)-1 and -2, West Nile virus, *Treponema pallidum* (syphilis), *Trypanosoma cruzi* (Chagas' disease), and cytomegalovirus (CMV).[30] Not every test is performed everywhere and for every unit (eg, *Trypanosoma cruzi* and CMV tests). Other infective threats to blood safety not currently tested for include *Babesia*; *Plasmodium* (malaria); prions (Creutzfeldt-Jakob disease, new variant [nvCJD]); hepatitis A virus; human herpesvirus 8; and chikungunya virus.[25] Various methods of pathogen inactivation (without the need for specific testing) are under investigation and some have been implemented, but their efficacy and effect on the quality of the blood products remain to be determined.[31]

Current estimated risks of infection per RBC unit range from 1 in 100,000 to 1 in 400,000 for HBV; 1 in 1.6 million to 1 in 3.1 million for HCV; 1 in 1.4 million to 1 in 4.7 million for HIV; and 1 in 500,000 to 1 in 3 million for HTLV.[4,26,32–34] The risk of acquiring malaria through allogeneic transfusion is estimated at 1 in 4 million units. There have been seven cases of Chagas' disease and four cases of nvCJD confirmed to be transmitted through transfusions.[35–36] Finally, bacterial contamination is present in 1 in 28,000 to 1 in 143,000 units of RBCs, but it is much more common in platelets (1/2000–1/8000 units).[4,26,32–34] Of note, bacterial infections remain the leading cause of mortality due to transfusion-transmitted infections, accounting for 17% to 22% of all such cases.[37] The most common organisms in RBC units include *Yersinia enterocolitica*, *Pseudomonas spp.*, and *Serratia spp.*[37] Other potential hazards include Epstein-Barr virus, leishmaniasis, Lyme disease, brucellosis, and human herpesviruses. Despite a relatively high rate of viremia in blood donors, only a few cases of anemia due to transfusion-transmitted parvovirus B19 have been reported.[38] Hepatitis G virus, SEN virus, and transfusion-transmitted virus are other infective agents commonly found in blood (1–2/100 donations), but their significance is presently unknown.[39] Specific patient populations may be at increased risk, as exemplified by the susceptibility of seronegative immunosuppressed patients to CMV, which mandates the use of leukoreduced blood products from seronegative donors for these patients. It has been suggested that leukocyte reduction may reduce the risk of other transfusion-transmitted infections, including other herpesviruses, bacteria, and protozoa.[40]

Noninfectious risks of transfusion (see **Table 1**) often receive less publicity compared with the infectious risks, but they are far more common and exceed the infectious risks by many factors when the total burden of disease (complications) is considered: the aggregate risk of transmission of major viral threads (ie, HBV, HCV, HIV, and HTLV) by way of transfusion is estimated at approximately 1 in 30,000 units or less. Moreover, not every transmission leads to a full-blown infection, and therefore, the rate of clinically significant infections may be even lower.[38,41] In contrast, a single noninfectious complication—transfusion-related acute lung injury [TRALI]—is estimated to occur in 1 out of every 5000 units of blood transfused, and possibly even more commonly because it is often unrecognized or underreported.[42] Noninfectious risks can be grouped under immunologic and nonimmunologic complications (see **Table 1**). It should be noted that this classification is somewhat arbitrary because many nonimmunologic reactions also have some immunologic components.

Allogeneic transfusion can have suppressive and stimulatory effects on the immune system. It was noticed in the 1960s that blood transfusion could prolong survival of allografts in animal models; in the 1970s, similar results were confirmed in patients receiving cadaver kidney transplantation following multiple allogeneic blood transfusions.[43] Despite the seemingly beneficial effects of transplantation in women who have multiple miscarriages, transfusion-related immunomodulation has been also reported to be associated with an increased rate of cancer recurrence and postoperative infection in some observational studies; these associations are still being debated. Leukocytes appear to play the major role in transfusion-related immunomodulation.[44,45]

New antigen variants introduced into the body through allogeneic transfusion can stimulate the immune system to produce alloantibodies against blood cells (alloimmunization). RBC alloimmunization is one of the most frequent complications following transfusion and is more common in multiple-transfused patients (eg, patients who have sickle cell anemia).[46] Unlike long-recognized major blood groups, a large number of heterogeneous antigens (eg, various HLA classes) can cause alloimmunization. Transfusion of RBCs with such an antigen to a patient who has preformed alloantibodies against that antigen (eg, due to sensitization in previous transfusions) can result in hemolytic reactions. These so-called "delayed hemolytic reactions" occur in aproximately one in 1000 to one in 9000 RBC units transfused, as opposed to acute hemolytic reactions due to transfusion of ABO-incompatible blood, which are less frequent but do not require previous exposure.[22,38,44,45] Allergic transfusion complications range form mild reactions such as urticaria (occurring in 8% of transfusions) to severe deadly anaphylactic shock in immunoglobulin A–deficient patients.[47]

Transfusion-associated graft-versus-host disease (TA-GVHD) is another rare immunologic complication of transfusion in which immunocompetent, HLA-incompatible donor lymphocytes are transfused to a recipient who is immunologically incapable of eliminating them, and these cells elicit an immune response against host cells. Patients at risk of TA-GVHD include those who have cell-mediated immunodeficiencies, recipients of bone marrow transplants, and patients receiving immunosuppressive therapy. Use of irradiated blood components can eliminate the risk of TA-GVHD and should be considered in susceptible patients.[48] The condition is rare, is difficult to treat, and has a 90% mortality.[38]

Among the nonimmunologic transfusion risks, transfusion errors are estimated to occur in one in 12,000 units transfused.[49] The most obvious error is transfusion of ABO-incompatible blood, which can result in an immediate hemolytic reaction, and it remains a leading cause of fatal transfusion reactions. Other transfusion errors include erroneous transfusion of units that have tested positive for an infection and the issuance of blood for patients for whom autologous blood is available.[49]

TRALI is characterized by acute-onset respiratory distress, bilateral pulmonary edema, fever, tachycardia, and hypotension in the presence of normal cardiac function occurring within 6 hours following transfusion. TRALI can be confused with other transfusion-related or unrelated disorders and is believed to be frequently misdiagnosed and underreported.[42] Its etiology is multifactorial and likely to be related to the reaction of antibodies present in donor blood with antigens of recipient's neutrophils, leading to increased permeability of the pulmonary vessels.[44] Despite a clinical presentation similar to acute respiratory distress syndrome (ARDS), TRALI is usually transient and its mortality rate is lower at approximately 5% to 10%.[42] Transfusion-associated circulatory overload (TACO) is another complication of transfusion and presents with pulmonary edema and respiratory distress. Unlike TRALI, which is associated with increased vascular permeability, pulmonary edema in TACO is caused by increased central venous pressure and pulmonary blood volume resulting in fluid extravasation into alveolar space. TACO is estimated to occur in 1 in 3000 to as many as one in 10 transfusions depending on the patient population and definition. Distinguishing TRALI from TACO can pose a challenge; often, varying degrees of both are present together.[50]

Febrile nonhemolytic transfusion reaction is the most common cause of transfusion-associated fever, occurring in 0.1% to 1% of RBC transfusions.[38] Leukoreduction can decrease the incidence of this complication.[51] Other causes of transfusion-associated fever (eg, hemolytic reactions, bacterial contamination, TRALI) are more serious and should be considered in febrile patients.

After removal from the body and with the added effect of storage, RBCs undergo changes (many irreversible) that adversely affect their viability and function. These adverse changes include oxidation and rearrangement of lipids, loss of proteins, and depletion of ATP and 2,3-diphosphoglycerate. In storage, RBCs continuously lose their membrane through shedding vesicles and become rigid.[52,53] Moreover, during storage, bioactive by-products and ions (eg, Hb, lipids, and potassium)—some with proinflammatory effects—are released from RBCs and accumulate in blood units whereby they can cause adverse reactions in a recipient.[54] These changes are collectively called "storage lesion."[52–54] Transfusion of blood that is stored for prolonged periods (but still within the currently accepted maximum allowed storage time of 42 days) has been linked to increased risk of complications and reduced survival in patients undergoing cardiac surgery and in other patient populations.[52–55] Some studies suggest that leukodepletion may improve the quality of stored blood products and help reduce adverse outcomes.[54]

When discussing the risks of transfusion, attention is paid primarily to the recipients of blood. It should be noted, however, that blood donation is not free of risk, and donors may experience adverse reactions and complications related to donating blood. Complications include presyncopeal symptoms, loss of consciousness, hematomas, chest pain, and allergic reactions. The incidence of donation-related complications is higher in younger donors, first-time donors, and women.[56]

Worsening of outcomes in transfused patients is a theme repeatedly observed in studies comparing transfused with nontransfused patients in various settings and populations, including critically ill patients, elderly patients, cardiac surgery cases, trauma patients, orthopedic surgical cases, and patients who have acute coronary syndrome. In these studies, patients receiving allogeneic transfusions have had higher mortality rates, higher risk of ICU admission, longer hospital and ICU stays, higher postoperative infection rates, higher risk of developing ARDS, longer time to ambulation, higher incidence of atrial fibrillation, and higher risk of ischemic outcomes compared with nontransfused cohorts (**Table 2**).[18,19,21,57–79] One caveat of most of these studies is the uncontrolled methodology and observational nature of the study. Designing a randomized controlled trial with a no-transfusion arm poses many ethical and recruitment challenges. Using the data from patients refusing allogeneic transfusions as the control arm is an option, but those participating cannot be randomized and other approaches for matching are needed. Nonetheless, randomized controlled trials comparing restrictive with liberal transfusion strategies in critically ill patients have shown that in most of the patients, outcomes of restrictively transfused patients are at least similar to their liberally transfused counterparts, if not better.[80,81]

When considering the generally unfavorable outcomes associated with allogeneic transfusion in the studies, it should be remembered that every patient has a unique oxygen delivery and consumption status and that tolerance for anemia differs among different cases. In other words, each study may include patients who have varying levels of Hb (although as discussed earlier, mere Hb level is not an accurate indicator of oxygen delivery and consumption), and some of these patients may indeed benefit from transfusion. For example, it has been reported that blood transfusion can lower the short-term mortality rate in elderly patients who have myocardial infarction and who have a hematocrit of 33 or less on admission.[71] Although several limitations (eg, retrospective nature, potential baseline differences between the groups, and consideration of admission hematocrit as opposed to more relevant nadir hematocrit

Table 2
Outcomes of transfusion

Setting/Population	Outcomes Associated with Transfusion	Study
Cardiac surgery	Increased mortality rate; longer ICU stay	Leal-Noval et al, 2001[57]
	Higher incidence of bacterial infection	Chelemer et al, 2002[58]
	Increased 5-year mortality rate; higher incidence of serious postoperative infections	Engoren et al, 2002[59]
	Higher risk of developing AF	Koch et al, 2006[60]
	Increased mortality rate; higher risk of renal failure, prolonged respiratory support, serious infection, cardiac complications, and neurologic events	Koch et al, 2006[61]
	Reduced long-term survival	Koch et al, 2006[62]
	Delayed discharge from hospital; higher risk of death within 30 d; higher risk of infection; higher risk of ischemia	Murphy et al, 2007[18]
Colorectal surgery	Higher risk of postoperative infection and intra-abdominal sepsis	Chang et al, 2000[63]
ICU/critically ill patients	Increased overall and ICU 14-d mortality rate; higher 28-d mortality rate	Vincent et al, 2002[64]
	Increased mortality rate; longer length of stay; more total number of complications	Corwin et al, 2004[65]
	Increased mortality rate; higher risk of developing ARDS	Gong et al, 2005[66]
	Higher incidence of bloodstream infections	Shorr et al, 2005[67]
	Higher risk of nosocomial infection	Taylor et al, 2006[68]
	Higher risk of developing ARDS	Zilberberg et al, 2007[69]
	Increased hospital mortality rate; prolonged hospital stay	Zilberberg et al, 2008[70]
Myocardial infarction/ischemia	Increased 30-d mortality rate if hematocrit on admission was >36%	Wu et al, 2001[71]
	Increased 30-d mortality	Rao et al, 2004[19]
	Increased risk of in-hospital mortality	Jani et al, 2007[21]
Orthopedics	Higher risk of bacterial infection; higher risk of pneumonia	Carson et al, 1999[72]
	Higher risk of infection	Innerhofer et al, 2005[73]
	Longer time to ambulation; longer length of stay	Weber et al, 2005[74]
Subarachnoid hemorrhage	Higher risk of vasospasm and poor outcome	Smith et al, 2004[75]
Trauma	Higher risk of developing infection	Claridge et al, 2002[76]
	Increased mortality rate; higher risk of ICU admission; longer ICU and hospital length of stay	Malone et al, 2003[77]
	Increased mortality rate; higher risk of ICU admission; higher incidence of SIRS	Dunne et al, 2004[78]
	Increased mortality rate; higher risk of developing ARDS	Silverboard et al, 2005[79]

Abbreviations: AF, atrial fibrillation; SIRS, systemic inflammatory response syndrome.

levels)[82] negatively affect the reliability of the observations of this study,[71] the results point to the fact that every transfusion decision is, in essence, a risk/benefit analysis. Allogeneic blood transfusions are associated with many risks, but in specific (and limited) circumstances, their benefits outweigh the risks. Under most circumstances, the benefit-to-risk ratio of allogeneic blood transfusions is not favorable, and such transfusions should be avoided or replaced by alternatives.

COSTS OF TRANSFUSION

The price tag of a unit of allogeneic RBCs represents a gross understatement of the true cost of blood. What most health care providers see as the act of transfusion (ie, ordering blood and infusing it) is just the tip of the iceberg of the numerous procedures required to procure, process, store, and distribute blood. In addition, dealing with side effects and the direct and indirect consequences of transfusion is an added cost that is usually ignored. An example is the compensation paid to the recipients of HIV-contaminated transfusions totaling billions of dollars in many countries.[83]

A number of studies have tried to estimate the true cost of blood by accounting for often-forgotten steps involved.[84] The results vary depending on the methodology of the studies, the extent and depth of the steps covered, and the perspective of the investigators, and range from $326 to $850 per unit of RBCs (adjusted for 2007 value).[85–86] It should be remembered that these figures reflect the cost of regular blood units at the time the studies were performed (ie, in the 1990s), and additional processing (eg, irradiation, deglycerolization) is associated with added costs. Another additional process, leukoreduction, has become a universal practice in many countries and its costs have not been incorporated in these figures. Finally, today's added safety of the blood supply from infectious risks has been achieved at the expense of more laborious and complicated screening and testing procedures. Although it may appear at first glance that these added costs are worth the reduced risk, it is enlightening to point out that each quality-adjusted life year (QALY) saved by adding more sensitive HIV nucleic acid testing to the serologic screening on donated blood comes at an estimated cost of over $1.5 million.[87] At the individual patient level, we may be willing to pay extra to feel safer against HIV; however, nucleic acid testing falls considerably short of the generally accepted cost-effectiveness bar set at $50,000 to $80,000 per QALY for health care interventions.[84] It is no wonder that this has been called the "price of fear."[88]

Comprehensive efforts to capture the true cost of blood are underway. The first Cost-of-Blood Consensus Conference (COBCON I) was convened by the Society for the Advancement of Blood Management (www.SABM.org) in 2003 to develop an all-inclusive model.[83] The result was a nine-step process flow model encompassing cost elements associated with blood collection (ie, donor recruitment and qualification, blood collection, blood processing and laboratory testing, blood disposal and donor notification [in case of positive test results], and blood storage and transport) and transfusion services (ie, blood service inventory and storage, pretransfusion preparation, transfusion administration and follow-up, and tracking of long-term outcomes). Societal cost elements (eg, donors' and recipients' loss of productivity) were also included. In total, over 250 cost-incurring steps were identified in the transfusion process. It was concluded that the true cost of blood was far greater than what was charged by the blood collection agencies in the United States.[83]

A newer model based on activity-based costing has been developed and efforts are underway to outline the transfusion process by breaking it into individual activities (COBCON II).[83] Preliminary results based on only a few steps of the process already indicate an estimated cost of over $1400 per transfused unit.[84] Although the final esti-mated cost is expected to be significantly higher, even the current incomplete figure is twice as much as the highest previous estimate of the cost of blood. Considering the 14 million blood units transfused annually in the United States,[89] the difference amounts to $10 billion.

The true annual burden of transfusion on health care expenditure is expected to be tens of billion dollars. When all the cost elements involved in transfusion are accounted for, a more accurate picture will become available; however, even the currently avail-able limited data are more than sufficient to provide us with an idea of the magnitude of the costs involved. Appreciation of the true cost of blood transfusions will undoubtedly promote justified used of transfusion and its alternatives.[84]

WHEN BLOOD IS NOT AN OPTION

In addition to blood units being costly, they are difficult to procure, prepare, transport, and store. Blood supply in the Unite States and many developed nations is based on voluntary donations as recommended by 28th World Health Assembly over 3 decades ago.[90] An aging population and more restrictive screening criteria has resulted in a shrinking pool of donors and has limited the supply. Currently, it is estimated that 111 million individuals in the United States are eligible to donate blood.[91] The number of actual donors, however, is significantly smaller. A survey of blood supply and demand in the United States indicated that although blood donation increased by 10.4% from 1999 to 2001, transfusion increased by 12.2%, reducing the margin between transfusion demand and supply from 9.1% to 7.9% of the total supply. It should be noted that the year 2001 witnessed a dramatic increase in donations following the September 11 terrorist attacks, and this margin is likely to be much nar-rower today.[92] If the current trend of increasing demand and diminishing supply continues (which is the likely scenario, as indicated by the reluctance of the "new generation" to donate blood),[93] the result will be an imminent shortage of blood components at the national level.

Given the complicated nature of processing, transportation, and storage of blood, local shortages are far more likely to happen. The delicate chain of supply can easily be disrupted and overwhelmed by disasters, conflicts, and mass casualty events.[94,95] Due to the increased stress and workload during such events, the probability of trans-fusion errors is also likely to increase.[94] More commonly, as can be seen in everyday accidents and incidences in remote areas, blood might simply not be available at the field for trauma victims. The same logistic limitations are present in combat zones. Transfusion of unscreened fresh whole blood is a controversial practice recognized by the United States military for patients who have life-threatening traumatic injuries and can expose recipients to increased risk of infection.[96]

Unlike developed countries, in many regions of the world, providing access to a safe blood supply remains a major challenge.[97–98] Many developing nations still rely largely on remunerated repeat donors who often carry a higher risk of infections.[99] Due to limited resources, donated blood cannot be and is not tested as rigorously as in devel-oped countries: from 2001 to 2002, 6 million required tests for the markers of the four main transfusion-transmitted infections (HIV, HBV, HCV, and syphilis) were not per-formed on donated blood units.[100] The result is a staggering high incidence of trans-fusion-transmitted infections in less developed nations (eg, 5%–15% of total new HIV infections are transmitted through transfusions).[99]

In addition to logistic constraints affecting the availability of safe blood, there are certain situations in which allogeneic transfusions are not acceptable despite availability. Some patients refuse allogeneic blood products due to religious reasons.[101] Blood transfusion is not an option in some cases of autoimmune hemolytic anemia because the transfused RBCs are targeted and lysed by the immune system. In these cases and in circumstances of unavailability of blood, the use of alternatives to transfusion is often the only option to save the lives of severely anemic patients.

SUMMARY

Chronic anemia is an independent predictor of mortality and morbidity, and it should be screened for, properly diagnosed, and treated.[102] Several adaptive mechanisms are activated in response to anemia to maintain oxygen delivery to the tissues. As a result, significant drops in Hb level can be well tolerated in most patients. In fact, in most cases, anemia is much better tolerated by patients than by their attending physicians who rush to order blood at first drop of Hb. As [Hb] decreases below a critical level, tissue oxygen consumption is compromised and signs of ischemia may appear. At this point, aggressive treatments to improve the oxygen-delivery capacity of blood are required.

Allogeneic blood transfusions are associated with a long list of infectious and noninfectious risks. A multitude of studies have demonstrated worse outcomes in patients who have been transfused, and randomized trials indicate that outcomes in restrictively transfused patients are similar to or better than outcomes in liberally transfused cases. Blood is costly and it cannot be made available or used in many situations. Recommended global strategies include restricting allogeneic blood transfusions and limiting their use to specific patients who are expected to benefit from transfusion based on objective criteria.

Alternatives to transfusion that can perform the oxygen-carrying function of blood without all the risks associated with transfusion are promising options, and they can be life-saving agents in many patients for whom blood is not available or not an option. Safer and more effective alternatives to blood are warranted to replace allogeneic blood altogether in the (limited) indications of transfusion. Elimination of infectious risks, immunologic interactions, compatibility issues, and specific storage requirements are just some of the incentives of developing such modalities. This is an exciting field with enormous potential to save millions of lives and change the face of transfusion medicine forever. Soon, blood will return to its place next to the three other humors in the books of history and we will begin using real therapeutic agents with defined safety and efficacy profiles specifically developed for transporting oxygen to tissues.

ACKNOWLEDGMENTS

The authors thank Mazyar Javidroozi, MD, for his contribution to the editing of this manuscript. He declares no conflict of interests.

REFERENCES

1. Alberts B, Johnson A, Lewis J, et al. Molecular biology of the cell. 4th edition. New York: Garland Science; 2002. p. 3–45.
2. Hardison RC. A brief history of hemoglobins: plant, animal, protist, and bacteria. Proc Natl Acad Sci U S A 1996;93(12):5675–9.
3. Shander A. Anemia in the critically ill. Crit Care Clin 2004;20(2):159–78.

4. Madjdpour C, Spahn DR, Weiskopf RB. Anemia and perioperative red blood cell transfusion: a matter of tolerance. Crit Care Med 2006;34(Suppl 5): S102–8.

5. Marshall JC. Transfusion trigger: when to transfuse? Crit Care 2004;8(Suppl 2): S31–3.

6. Weiskopf RB, Viele MK, Feiner J, et al. Human cardiovascular and metabolic response to acute, severe isovolemic anemia. JAMA 1998;279(3):217–21.

7. Fowler NO, Holmes JC. Blood viscosity and cardiac output in acute experimental anemia. J Appl Physiol 1975;39(3):453–6.

8. Habler OP, Kleen MS, Podtschaske AH, et al. The effect of acute normovolemic hemodilution (ANH) on myocardial contractility in anesthetized dogs. Anesth Analg 1996;83(3):451–8.

9. Barbee JH, Cokelet GR. The Fahraeus effect. Microvasc Res 1971;3(1):6–16.

10. Chapler CK, Cain SM. The physiologic reserve in oxygen carrying capacity: studies in experimental hemodilution. Can J Physiol Pharmacol 1986;64(1):7–12.

11. Morisaki H, Sibbald WJ. Tissue oxygen delivery and the microcirculation. Crit Care Clin 2004;20(2):213–23.

12. Hebert PC, Van der Linden P, Biro G, et al. Physiologic aspects of anemia. Crit Care Clin 2004;20(2):187–212.

13. van Bommel J, Siegemund M, Henny ChP, et al. Heart, kidney, and intestine have different tolerances for anemia. Transl Res 2008;151(2):110–7.

14. Cabrales P, Tsai AG, Intaglietta M. Is resuscitation from hemorrhagic shock limited by blood oxygen-carrying capacity or blood viscosity? Shock 2007; 27(4):380–9.

15. Ickx BE, Rigolet M, Van Der Linden PJ. Cardiovascular and metabolic response to acute normovolemic anemia. Effects of anesthesia. Anesthesiology 2000; 93(4):1011–6.

16. Spahn DR, Seifert B, Pasch T, et al. Haemodilution tolerance in patients with mitral regurgitation. Anaesthesia 1998;53(1):20–4.

17. Roseberg B, Wulff K. Hemodynamics following normovolemic hemodilution in elderly patients. Acta Anaesthesiol Scand 1981;25(5):402–6.

18. Murphy GJ, Reeves BC, Rogers CA, et al. Increased mortality, postoperative morbidity, and cost after red blood cell transfusion in patients having cardiac surgery. Circulation 2007;116(22):2544–52.

19. Rao SV, Jollis JG, Harrington RA, et al. Relationship of blood transfusion and clinical outcomes in patients with acute coronary syndromes. JAMA 2004; 292(13):1555–62.

20. Gerber DR. Transfusion of packed red blood cells in patients with ischemic heart disease. Crit Care Med 2008;36(4):1068–74.

21. Jani SM, Smith DE, Share D, et al. Blood transfusion and in-hospital outcomes in anemic patients with myocardial infarction undergoing percutaneous coronary intervention. Clin Cardiol 2007;30(10 Suppl 2):II49–56.

22. Madjdpour C, Heindl V, Spahn DR. Risks, benefits, alternatives and indications of allogenic blood transfusions. Minerva Anestesiol 2006;72(5):283–98.

23. Hébert PC, McDonald BJ, Tinmouth A. Clinical consequences of anemia and red cell transfusion in the critically ill. Crit Care Clin 2004;20(2):225–35.

24. Goodnough LT. Transfusion triggers. Surgery 2007;142(Suppl 4):S67–70.

25. Shander A, Goodnough LT. Update on transfusion medicine. Pharmacotherapy 2007;27(9 Pt 2):57S–68S.

26. Dodd RY. Current risk for transfusion transmitted infections. Curr Opin Hematol 2007;14(6):671–6.

27. Becker JL. Vector-borne illnesses and the safety of the blood supply. Curr Hematol Rep 2003;2(6):511–7.
28. Arguin PM, Singleton J, Rotz LD, et al. An investigation into the possibility of transmission of tick-borne pathogens via blood transfusion. Transfusion-Associated Tick-Borne Illness Task Force. Transfusion 1999;39(8):828–33.
29. Shander A. Emerging risks and outcomes of blood transfusion in surgery. Semin Hematol 2004;41(1 Suppl 1):117–24.
30. Klein HG. Pathogen inactivation technology: cleansing the blood supply. J Intern Med 2005;257(3):224–37.
31. Webert KE, Cserti CM, Hannon J, et al. Proceedings of a Consensus Conference: pathogen inactivation-making decisions about new technologies. Transfus Med Rev 2008;22(1):1–34.
32. Busch MP, Kleinman SH, Nemo GJ. Current and emerging infectious risks of blood transfusions. JAMA 2003;289(8):959–62.
33. Klein HG, Spahn DR, Carson JL. Red blood cell transfusion in clinical practice. Lancet 20074;370(9585):415–426.
34. Brown P. Creutzfeldt-Jakob disease: reflections on the risk from blood product therapy. Haemophilia 2007;13(Suppl 5):33–40.
35. Goodnough LT, Brecher ME, Kanter MH, et al. Transfusion medicine. First of two parts–blood transfusion. N Engl J Med 1999;340(6):438–47.
36. Editorial team. Fourth case of transfusion-associated vCJD infection in the United Kingdom. Euro Surveill 200718;12(1):E070118.4
37. Wagner SJ. Transfusion-transmitted bacterial infection: risks, sources and interventions. Vox Sang 2004;86(3):157–63.
38. Kleinman S, Chan P, Robillard P. Risks associated with transfusion of cellular blood components in Canada. Transfus Med Rev 2003;17(2):120–62.
39. Canadian Paediatric Society. Transfusion and risk of infection in Canada: Update 2006. Can J Infect Dis Med Microbiol 2006;17(2):103–7.
40. Cervia JS, Wenz B, Ortolano GA. Leukocyte reduction's role in the attenuation of infection risks among transfusion recipients. Clin Infect Dis 2007;45(8):1008–13.
41. Schreiber GB, Busch MP, Kleinman SH, Korelitz JJ. The risk of transfusion-transmitted viral infections. The Retrovirus Epidemiology Donor Study. N Engl J Med 1996;334(26):1685–90.
42. Shander A, Popovsky MA. Understanding the consequences of transfusion-related acute lung injury. Chest 2005;128(5 Suppl 2):598S–604S.
43. Waanders MM, Roelen DL, Brand A, et al. The putative mechanism of the immunomodulating effect of HLA-DR shared allogeneic blood transfusions on the alloimmune response. Transfus Med Rev 2005;19(4):281–7.
44. Goodnough LT. Risks of blood transfusion. Anesthesiol Clin North America 2005;23(2):241–52, v.
45. Goodnough LT. Risks of blood transfusion. Crit Care Med 2003;31(12 Suppl):S678–86.
46. Bauer MP, Wiersum-Osselton J, Schipperus M, et al. Clinical predictors of alloimmunization after red blood cell transfusion. Transfusion 2007;47(11):2066–71.
47. Klein HG, Spahn DR, Carson JL. Red blood cell transfusion in clinical practice. Lancet 2007;370(9585):415–26.
48. Anderson K. Broadening the spectrum of patient groups at risk for transfusion-associated GVHD: implications for universal irradiation of cellular blood components. Transfusion 2003;43(12):1652–4.
49. Linden JV, Paul B, Dressler KP. A report of 104 transfusion errors in New York State. Transfusion 1992;32(7):601–6.

50. Skeate RC, Eastlund T. Distinguishing between transfusion related acute lung injury and transfusion associated circulatory overload. Curr Opin Hematol 2007;14(6):682–7.

51. King KE, Shirey RS, Thoman SK, et al. Universal leukoreduction decreases the incidence of febrile nonhemolytic transfusion reactions to RBCs. Transfusion 2004;44(1):25–9.

52. Tinmouth A, Fergusson D, Yee IC, et al. ABLE Investigators; Canadian Critical Care Trials Group. Clinical consequences of red cell storage in the critically ill. Transfusion 2006;46(11):2014–27.

53. Kriebardis AG, Antonelou MH, Stamoulis KE, et al. Storage-dependent remodeling of the red blood cell membrane is associated with increased immunoglobulin G binding, lipid raft rearrangement, and caspase activation. Transfusion 2007; 47(7):1212–20.

54. Ho J, Sibbald WJ, Chin-Yee IH. Effects of storage on efficacy of red cell transfusion: when is it not safe? Crit Care Med 2003;31(12 Suppl):S687–97.

55. Koch CG, Li L, Sessler DI, et al. Duration of red-cell storage and complications after cardiac surgery. N Engl J Med 2008;358(12):1229–39.

56. Eder AF, Hillyer CD, Dy BA, et al. Adverse reactions to allogeneic whole blood donation by 16- and 17-year-olds. JAMA 2008;299(19):2279–86.

57. Leal-Noval SR, Rincón-Ferrari MD, García-Curiel A, et al. Transfusion of blood components and postoperative infection in patients undergoing cardiac surgery. Chest 2001;119(5):1461–8.

58. Chelemer SB, Prato BS, Cox PM Jr, et al. Association of bacterial infection and red blood cell transfusion after coronary artery bypass surgery. Ann Thorac Surg 2002;73(1):138–42.

59. Engoren MC, Habib RH, Zacharias A, et al. Effect of blood transfusion on long-term survival after cardiac operation. Ann Thorac Surg 2002;74(4):1180–6.

60. Koch CG, Li L, Van Wagoner DR, et al. Red cell transfusion is associated with an increased risk for postoperative atrial fibrillation. Ann Thorac Surg 2006;82(5): 1747–56.

61. Koch CG, Li L, Duncan AI, et al. Morbidity and mortality risk associated with red blood cell and blood-component transfusion in isolated coronary artery bypass grafting. Crit Care Med 2006;34(6):1608–16.

62. Koch CG, Li L, Duncan AI, et al. Transfusion in coronary artery bypass grafting is associated with reduced long-term survival. Ann Thorac Surg 2006;81(5):1650–7.

63. Chang H, Hall GA, Geerts WH, et al. Allogeneic red blood cell transfusion is an independent risk factor for the development of postoperative bacterial infection. Vox Sang 2000;78(1):13–8.

64. Vincent JL, Baron JF, Reinhart K, et al. ABC (Anemia and Blood Transfusion in Critical Care) Investigators. Anemia and blood transfusion in critically ill patients. JAMA 2002;288(12):1499–507.

65. Corwin HL, Gettinger A, Pearl RG, et al. The CRIT Study: Anemia and blood transfusion in the critically ill–current clinical practice in the United States. Crit Care Med 2004;32(1):39–52.

66. Gong MN, Thompson BT, Williams P, et al. Clinical predictors of and mortality in acute respiratory distress syndrome: potential role of red cell transfusion. Crit Care Med 2005;33(6):1191–8.

67. Shorr AF, Jackson WL, Kelly KM, et al. Transfusion practice and blood stream infections in critically ill patients. Chest 2005;127(5):1722–8.

68. Taylor RW, O'Brien J, Trottier SJ, et al. Red blood cell transfusions and nosocomial infections in critically ill patients. Crit Care Med 2006;34(9):2302–8.

69. Zilberberg MD, Carter C, Lefebvre P, et al. Red blood cell transfusions and the risk of acute respiratory distress syndrome among the critically ill: a cohort study. Crit Care 2007;11(3):R63.
70. Zilberberg MD, Stern LS, Wiederkehr DP, et al. Anemia, transfusions and hospital outcomes among critically ill patients on prolonged acute mechanical ventilation: a retrospective cohort study. Crit Care 2008;12(2):R60.
71. Wu WC, Rathore SS, Wang Y, et al. Blood transfusion in elderly patients with acute myocardial infarction. N Engl J Med 2001;345(17):1230–6.
72. Carson JL, Altman DG, Duff A, et al. Risk of bacterial infection associated with allogeneic blood transfusion among patients undergoing hip fracture repair. Transfusion 1999;39(7):694–700.
73. nnerhofer P, Klingler A, Klimmer C, et al. Risk for postoperative infection after transfusion of white blood cell-filtered allogeneic or autologous blood components in orthopedic patients undergoing primary arthroplasty. Transfusion 2005;45(1):103–10.
74. Weber EW, Slappendel R, Prins MH, et al. Perioperative blood transfusions and delayed wound healing after hip replacement surgery: effects on duration of hospitalization. Anesth Analg 2005;100(5):1416–21.
75. Smith MJ, Le Roux PD, Elliott JP, et al. Blood transfusion and increased risk for vasospasm and poor outcome after subarachnoid hemorrhage. J Neurosurg 2004;101(1):1–7.
76. Claridge JA, Sawyer RG, Schulman AM, et al. Blood transfusions correlate with infections in trauma patients in a dose-dependent manner. Am Surg 2002;68(7):566–72.
77. Malone DL, Dunne J, Tracy JK, et al. Blood transfusion, independent of shock severity, is associated with worse outcome in trauma. J Trauma 2003;54(5):898–905, discussion 905–7.
78. Dunne JR, Malone DL, Tracy JK, et al. Allogenic blood transfusion in the first 24 hours after trauma is associated with increased systemic inflammatory response syndrome (SIRS) and death. Surg Infect (Larchmt) 2004;5(4):395–404.
79. Silverboard H, Aisiku I, Martin GS, et al. The role of acute blood transfusion in the development of acute respiratory distress syndrome in patients with severe trauma. J Trauma 2005;59(3):717–23.
80. Hébert PC, Wells G, Blajchman MA, et al. A multicenter, randomized, controlled clinical trial of transfusion requirements in critical care. Transfusion Requirements in Critical Care Investigators, Canadian Critical Care Trials Group. N Engl J Med 1999;340(6):409–17.
81. Lacroix J, Hébert PC, Hutchison JS, et al. TRIPICU Investigators; Canadian Critical Care Trials Group; Pediatric Acute Lung Injury and Sepsis Investigators Network. Transfusion strategies for patients in pediatric intensive care units. N Engl J Med 2007;356(16):1609–19.
82. Goodnough LT, Bach RG. Anemia, transfusion, and mortality. N Engl J Med 2001;345(17):1272–4.
83. Participant of the Cost of Blood Consensus Conference, Charleston, SC, May 4–5, 2003. The cost of blood: multidisciplinary consensus conference for a standard methodology. Transfus Med Rev 2005;19(1):66–78.
84. Shander A, Hofmann A, Gombotz H, et al. Estimating the cost of blood: past, present, and future directions. Best Pract Res Clin Anaesthesiol 2007;21(2):271–89.
85. Etchason J, Petz L, Keeler E, et al. The cost effectiveness of preoperative autologous blood donations. N Engl J Med 1995;332(11):719–24.

86. Crémieux PY, Barrett B, Anderson K, et al. Cost of outpatient blood transfusion in cancer patients. J Clin Oncol 2000;18(14):2755–61.
87. Marshall DA, Kleinman SH, Wong JB, et al. Cost-effectiveness of nucleic acid test screening of volunteer blood donations for hepatitis B, hepatitis C and human immunodeficiency virus in the United States. Vox Sang 2004;86(1): 28–40.
88. Shander A. Financial and clinical outcomes associated with surgical bleeding complications. Surgery 2007;142(4 Suppl):S20–5.
89. Whitaker BI, Sullivan M, Henry R, United States Department of Health and Human Services. The 2005 Nationwide Blood Collection and Utilization Survey Report. 2005 [cited 05-29-2008]. Available at: http://www.hhs.gov/bloodsafety/ 2005NBCUS.pdf.
90. World Health Organization, Twenty-Eighth World Health Assembly, Geneva, 13–30 May 1975:WHA28.72 Utilization and Supply of Human Blood and Blood Products, World Health Organization, Geneva, 1975 [cited 05-29-2008]. Available at: http://www.who.int/bloodsafety/en/WHA28.72.pdf.
91. Riley W, Schwei M, McCullough J. The United States' potential blood donor pool: estimating the prevalence of donor-exclusion factors on the pool of potential donors. Transfusion 2007;47(7):1180–8.
92. Sullivan MT, Cotten R, Read EJ, et al. Blood collection and transfusion in the United States in 2001. Transfusion 2007;47(3):385–94.
93. Zou S, Musavi F, Notari EP 4th, et al. ARCNET Research Group. Changing age distribution of the blood donor population in the United States. Transfusion 2008; 48(2):251–7.
94. Dann EJ, Bonstein L, Arbov L, et al. Blood bank protocols for large-scale civilian casualty events: experience from terrorist bombing in Israel. Transfus Med 2007; 17(2):135–9.
95. Sandler SG, Ouellette GJ. Transportation and other blood system issues related to disasters: Washington, DC experience of September 11, 2002. Vox Sang 2002;83(Suppl 1):367–70.
96. Spinella PC, Perkins JG, Grathwohl KW, et al. 31st Combat Support Hospital Research Working Group. Risks associated with fresh whole blood and red blood cell transfusions in a combat support hospital. Crit Care Med 2007; 35(11):2576–81.
97. World Health Organization. Global Consultation on Universal Access to Safe Blood Transfusion. 9–11 June 2007, Ottawa, Canada [cited 05-29-2008]. Available at: http://www.who.int/bloodsafety/publications/Report_Global_Consultation_ Ottawa_2007.pdf.
98. Goodnough LT, Shander A, Brecher ME. Transfusion medicine: looking to the future. Lancet 2003;361(9352):161–9.
99. Bates I, Manyasi G, Medina Lara A. Reducing replacement donors in Sub-Saharan Africa: challenges and affordability. Transfus Med 2007;17(6):434–42.
100. World Health Organization. Global Database on Blood Safety Summary Report 2001–2. Geneva 2004 [cited 05-29-2008]. Available at. http://www.who.int/ bloodsafety/GDBS_Report_2001-2002.pdf.
101. Gohel MS, Bulbulia RA, Slim FJ, et al. How to approach major surgery where patients refuse blood transfusion (including Jehovah's Witnesses). Ann R Coll Surg Engl 2005;87(1):3–14.
102. Goodnough LT, Shander A, Spivak JL, et al. Detection, evaluation, and management of anemia in the elective surgical patient. Anesth Analg 2005;101(6): 1858–61.

Hemoglobin-based Oxygen Carriers: First, Second or Third Generation? Human or Bovine? Where are we Now?

Lena M. Napolitano, MD, FACS, FCCP, FCCM[a],*

KEYWORDS

- Hemoglobin-based oxygen carrier • HBOC • Intensive care
- Critical care • Blood transfusion • Hemoglobin

HEMOGLOBIN-BASED OXYGEN CARRIERS

The need for an alternative to allogeneic red blood cells (RBCs) for transfusion has been recognized for more than a century.[1–3] Concerns about the infectious and immunosuppressive risks of allogeneic blood products persist, and the increased disproportion between blood donation and consumption has reinforced the search for alternative erythrocyte transfusion strategies in recent years. The most serious motivation for the development of a blood substitute is the worldwide shortage of safe and viable allogeneic donor blood. A report on blood donations found that during 2001, 12.7% of hospitals reported cancellations of surgeries due to donor blood shortages and 18.9% reported shortages of blood for nonsurgical purposes.[4] In addition, the stress on the donated blood supply is projected to increase in the coming years.[5] Interestingly, even through blood transfusion has remained the standard of care, the efficacy and safety of allogeneic RBC therapy has never been rigorously tested via the clinical trial process.[6–8] Thus, comparing the safety and efficacy of a blood substitute, hemoglobin-based oxygen carriers (HBOCs), to the standard of care may prove to be difficult.

HBOCs are oxygen carriers that use purified human, animal, or recombinant hemoglobin (Hb) in a cell-free Hb preparation. They are infusible oxygen-carrying fluids that

---

[a] Department of Surgery, University of Michigan, Acute Care Surgery 1C340A-UH, 1500 E. Medical Center Drive, SPC 5033, Ann Arbor, MI 48109-5033, USA
* Surgical Critical Care and Trauma, University of Michigan, 1C340A-UH, 1500 E. Medical Center Drive, SPC 5033, Ann Arbor, MI 48109-5033.
E-mail address: lenan@umich.edu

Crit Care Clin 25 (2009) 279–301
doi:10.1016/j.ccc.2009.01.003
0749-0704/09/$ – see front matter © 2009 Published by Elsevier Inc.

have long shelf lives, have no need for refrigeration or cross-matching, could be in abundant supply, and are ideal for treating hemorrhagic shock in remote settings where blood is not available. Despite significant effort in the development of HBOCs, currently no such product is approved for use in North America or Europe, although several are in the clinical trial stage. One product is approved for use outside of the United States. Hemopure (polymerized bovine Hb, Biopure Corporation, Cambridge, Massachusetts) is approved for use in South Africa for adult surgery patients to treat acute anemia and reduce allogeneic blood use.[9]

Hb is a logical choice for an RBC substitute because of its high capacity to carry oxygen and its oncotic properties.[10] It also lacks the numerous and complex antigens of the RBC membrane, hence it is universally compatible. It is a robust molecule that withstands rigorous purification and viral inactivation processes, and it is stable under ordinary storage conditions.

The structure of Hb (**Fig. 1**) was determined in 1959 by Max Perutz, for which he was awarded a Nobel Prize. Human Hb is a 64-kDa tetrameric protein composed of two α subunits and two β-globin subunits that fold into a compact quaternary structure (α2β2). Each α and β-globin subunit contain an iron-heme group that binds to an oxygen molecule, allowing for transport. A fully saturated Hb molecule carries a maximum of four oxygen molecules. Environmental conditions such as paO_2, pH, temperature, and $paCO_2$ cause Hb to undergo conformational change from a high oxygen-affinity state to a lower oxygen-affinity state.

HBOCs are made by the lysis of RBCs releasing Hb molecules for purification and thorough sterilization and viral inactivation methods that are not possible with whole blood[11] or by recombinant technology. The three potential sources for Hb to make HBOCs are outdated human RBCs, bovine RBCs, and recombinant Hb (**Fig. 2**). Only 5% to 10% of donated allogeneic blood becomes outdated, and therefore, the quantity of Hb available from this source may not be sufficient for mass production of an HBOC.[12] Bovine Hb as a source for HBOCs has no quantity constraints.

Four main problems had to be overcome before Hb could be considered a serious candidate for a blood substitute. First, Hb in dilute solution is rapidly cleared by the

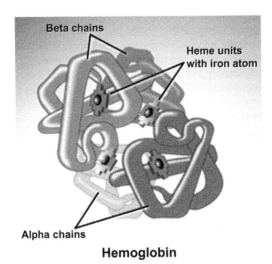

Hemoglobin

Fig. 1. Structure of Hb. (*From* www.chem.prudue.edu/courses/chm333/hemoglobin.jpg)

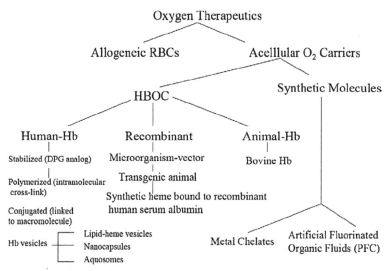

Fig. 2. Categories of RBC substitutes previously tested or currently in development. (*From* Ness PM, Cushing MM. Oxygen therapeutics. Arch Pathol Lab Med 2007;131:734–41; with permission.)

kidney because the tetrameric protein dissociates into smaller dimers and monomers. Second, dissociable tetramers and dimers with resultant free Hb bind with nitric oxide, inducing vasoconstriction and renal dysfunction (**Fig. 3**). Third, dilute Hb has a high affinity for oxygen. Fourth, even exceedingly small amounts of stromal (cell membrane) contaminants in Hb solutions appear to be toxic.[13]

Hemoglobin tetramer rapidly dissociates into dimers and monomers, gets filtered by the kidney, and causes potential damage to renal tubular cells. This issue was

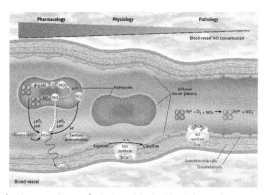

Fig. 3. A model of the interactions of nitric oxide (NO) with erythrocytes and cell-free Hb in an arterial blood vessel. The diagram illustrates the major processes regulating NO levels in blood vessels during pharmacologic NO delivery (*left*), under normal conditions (*center*), and under pathologic conditions, such as acute or chronic hemolysis (*right*). The overall blood vessel NO concentration is depicted by the thickness of the blue band above the vessel. Within the vessel, smooth muscle cells and a layer of endothelial cells are shown. Free Hb binds NO, resulting in vascular constriction, as depicted on the right side of the figure. (*From* Schechter AN, Gladwin MT. Hemoglobin and the paracrine and endocrine functions of nitric oxide. N Engl J Med 2003;348:1483–5; with permission.)

resolved by polymerization of the free Hb molecules (**Fig. 4**). This advance also led to reduced vasoreactivity via reduced nitric oxide binding. Ongoing advances have significantly improved HBOCs and resolved many of the prior problems that had been noted with the early HBOC solutions.

With the absence of problems such as nephrotoxicity, increased colloid osmotic pressure, and sudden renal clearance, modern HBOCs have shown their effectiveness and tolerability in numerous animal studies and several clinical studies. HBOCs can be infused without prior cross-matching and are now available as stable formulations with a long shelf life.[14] HBOCs may find application in differential indications, including as potent oxygen-delivering agents in addition to the globally recognized goal of being used as RBC substitutes in cases of significant bleeding.

Thus, eight different companies embarked on the development of an HBOC in the 1980s and 1990s. A number of HBOC products have been developed and have undergone preclinical and clinical testing (**Table 1**) as oxygen carriers and blood substitutes, although some have been discontinued related to safety issues. To date, only one product (Oxyglobin, polymerized bovine Hb, Biopure Corporation) is licensed for veterinary use and only one product (Hemopure) is approved for limited use in humans in South Africa when blood is not available.[15]

In March 2006, a workshop sponsored by the National Heart, Lung, and Blood Institute was convened to identify the role of basic science in clarifying the issues that are impeding progress in the development of HBOC solutions.[16] These discussions resulted in a consensus that, although HBOCs have shown clinical promise, various side effects have inhibited further development and regulatory approval, with cardiovascular events being of particular concern. Specific recommendations from this group included better understanding of the impact of HBOC infusion on human physiology, the need for development of rapid and noninvasive methods for the measurement of tissue oxygenation in human patients to better inform transfusion decisions, further investigation of the routes and consequences of Hb metabolism, optimization of clinical protocols for HBOC use, and assessment of the impact of HBOC formulation excipients.

The following section will review the history of HBOC development and specifically review the results of clinical trials of the more recent HBOCs.

FIRST-GENERATION HBOCs

The first-generation HBOCs were based on observations that cross-linking with, for example, glutaraldehyde, overcame Hb subunit dissociation and renal toxicity. Experience with these solutions showed that they can be vasoactive—sometimes increasing

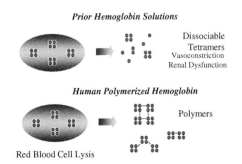

Fig. 4. PolyHeme-human Hb substitute.

Table 1
Status of HBOCs as of 2008

Product Class	Product	Company	Technology	Status
Cross-linked Hb	HemAssist (ααHb, DCLHb)	Baxter Corporation	Cross-linked Hb	Discontinued; safety;
		US Army	Cross-linked Hb	increased mortality
	rHb 1.1	Somatogen	rHb	Discontinued; safety; hypertension
	rHb 2.0	Baxter Corporation	rHb	Discontinued; safety
Polymerized Hb	PolyHeme	Northfield Laboratories Inc.	Glutaraldehyde, pyridoxal Hb	Phase III completed
	HBOC-201 (Hemopure)	Biopure Corporation	Glutaraldehyde bovine Hb	Phase III
	HemoLink	Hemosol Corporation	Polymerized Hb	Discontinued; safety; myocardial infarction
Conjugated Hb	PHP	Apex Bioscience	PEG–human Hb	Phase III; septic shock
	PEG-Hb	Enzon Inc. (Piscataway, NJ)	PEG–bovine Hb	Discontinued
	MalPEG-Hb	Sangart Inc.	PEG–human Hb	Phase III

Abbreviations: DCLHb, Diaspirin cross-linked Hb; MAL, Maleimide; PEG, Polyethylene glycol; PHP, Pyridoxylated Hb polyoxyethylene conjugate; rHb, Recombinant human Hb. *Adapted from* Winslow RM. Current status of oxygen carriers ("blood substitutes"): 2006. Vox Sang 2006;91(2):102–10.

blood pressure, sometimes decreasing tissue perfusion, and sometimes producing both actions. Clinical trials were disappointing because of unexpected toxicity.

A first-generation HBOC, diaspirin cross-linked Hb (DCLHb; HemAssist), was under development by Baxter Hemoglobin Therapeutics (Baxter International, Inc., Deerfield, Illinois) during the 1990s. This product had circumvented the safety concerns related to dimerization of the Hb tetramer by cross-linking the alpha chains chemically. Animal studies were promising.[17] The clinical studies performed with human cross-linked Hb (DCLHb) were stopped because of an increased rate of mortality in two clinical trials for patients who received DCLHb after stroke and multiple injury shock.[18,19] Additional studies in cases of cardiac and noncardiac surgery documented additional safety concerns, with early study termination related to serious adverse events.[20–22]

SECOND-GENERATION HBOCs

The second-generation HBOCs are based on a better understanding of the mechanisms of this vasoconstriction and specific modifications to reduce nitric oxide binding and resultant vasoconstriction. Four products have undergone recent clinical investigation (**Table 2**).

Three HBOC products (Hemopure, PolyHeme, MP4 (formerly Hemospan)) are currently in phase III clinical trials. The largest number of patients enrolled in HBOC clinical trials are in those investigating Hemopure and PolyHeme, and a comparison of the specific characteristics of these two HBOCs is delineated in **Table 3**.

Table 2
Four HBOCs in recent clinical trials

HBOC	Product	Company
Hemopure	Bovine Hb that is gluataraldehyde cross-linked to produce a polyHb	Biopure Corporation, Cambridge, Massachusetts
PolyHeme	Human Hb from donated human blood that is pyridoxylated to decrease the oxygen binding affinity and glutaraldehyde cross-linked to produce a polyHb	Northfield Laboratories Inc., Northfield, Illinois
HemoLink	Human Hb from donated human blood and O-raffinose cross-linked to produce a polyHb	Hemosol Corporation, Mississauga, Canada
MP4	PEG-conjugated human Hb	Sangart Inc., San Diego, California

Abbreviations: MP4, Maleimide PEG-Hb; PEG, Polyethylene glycol.

Hemopure

Hemopure (HBOC-201) is a polymerized form of bovine Hb with a p-50 of 30 mm Hg, which is closer to that of human Hb than stroma-free Hb. It has an intravascular half-life of from 8 hours to 23 hours and a shelf life of 36 months at room temperature. One unit of Hemopure contains 30 g of ultrapurified, chemically cross-linked Hb in 250 mL of a balanced salt solution.

When infused, these linked Hb molecules circulate in the plasma, are smaller and have a lower viscosity, and more readily release oxygen to tissues than those of allogeneic RBCs (**Fig. 5**).[23] Hemopure is compatible with all blood types and is purified through patented techniques that have been validated to remove infectious agents, including bacteria, viruses, prions, and other potential contaminants. A similar bovine Hb substitute is used in veterinary medicine as Oxyglobin.

Hemopure: Clinical Trials

Phase II and III studies with HBOC-201 have documented that infusion of HBOC-201 can avoid or reduce allogeneic blood transfusion needs for patients in specific perioperative settings.

Table 3
Characteristics of current HBOCs in phase III trials

Characteristic	Hemopure	PolyHeme	RBCs
Hb (g%)	13	10	13
Unit equivalent (g)	30	50	50
Molecular weight (> 64 k Da)	$\geq 95\%$	$\geq 99\%$	$\geq 100\%$
P_{50} (mm Hg)	38	29	26
Hill coefficient	1.4	1.7	2.7
Oncotic pressure (mm Hg)	25	23	25
Viscosity (cp)	1.3 cp	2.1 cp	(Whole blood = 5–10 cp)
Methemoglobin (%)	<10	<8	<1
Half-life	19 hours	24 hours	31 days
Shelf life at 4 C	≥ 3 years	≥ 1.5 years	42 days
Shelf life at 21 C	≥ 2 years	≥ 6 weeks	≥ 6 hours

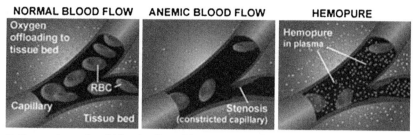

Fig. 5. Comparison of red blood cells and hemopure in plasma.

One clinical study evaluated HBOC-201 as a substitute for allogeneic RBC transfusion in patients undergoing elective infrarenal aortic operations (**Table 4**). In a single-blind, multicenter trial, 72 patients were prospectively randomized two-to-one to receive an HBOC-201 (n = 48) or allogeneic RBC (n = 24) at the time of the first transfusion decision, either during or after elective infrarenal aortic reconstruction. Patients randomized to the HBOC-201 group received 60 g of HBOC-201 for the initial transfusion and had the option to receive three more doses (30 g each) within 96 hours. In this group, any further blood requirement was met with allogeneic RBCs. Patients randomized to the allogeneic RBC group received only standard RBC transfusions. The efficacy analysis was a means of assessing the ability of the HBOC to eliminate the requirement for any allogeneic RBC transfusions from the time of randomization through 28 days later. The two treatment groups were comparable for all baseline characteristics. Although all patients in the allogeneic RBC group required at least one allogeneic RBC transfusion, 13 of 48 patients (27%; 95% confidence interval (CI), 15% to 42%) in the HBOC group did not require any allogeneic RBC transfusions. The only significant changes documented were a 15% increase in mean arterial pressure and a threefold peak increase in serum urea nitrogen concentration after HBOC transfusion. The complications were similar in both groups, with no allergic reactions. There were two perioperative deaths (8%) in the allogeneic RBC group and three perioperative deaths (6%) in the HBOC group ($P = 1.0$). This study concluded that the HBOC significantly eliminated the need for allogeneic RBC transfusion in 27% of patients undergoing infrarenal aortic reconstruction, but did not reduce the median

Table 4
Characteristics of Hemopure versus RBCs

Characteristics	Hemopure (HBOC-201)	RBCs
Storage	Room temperature (20–30 C)	Refrigerated
Shelf life	36 months	42 days
Preparations	Ready to use	Testing, typing, and cross-matching
Compatability	Universal	Type specific
Effectiveness	Immediate oxygen delivery	Dependant on length of storage
Purity	Processed to remove infectious agents	Tested and screened for infectious agents
Raw material	Bovine Hb abundant, controlled source	Limited availability, not controlled

allogeneic RBC requirement. HBOC transfusion was well tolerated and did not influence morbidity or mortality rates.[24]

A multicenter, randomized, single-blind trial (n = 81) compared HBOC-201 (n = 55) with an equivalent volume of Ringer's solution (n = 26) in surgical patients and evaluated the tolerability of a single intraoperative dose of HBOC-201. No deaths were reported; however a delayed dose-dependent increase in plasma methemoglobin concentration was noted. Intraoperative administration was well tolerated, up to a maximum of 245 g.[25]

Another randomized, double-blind, RBC-controlled, multicenter efficacy clinical trial (US Phase II Post-Cardiopulmonary Bypass Surgery Trial–1997) of the bovine Hb solution HBOC-201 (Hemopure) was performed in patients undergoing cardiac surgery and requiring blood transfusions. The object of this trial was to avoid RBC transfusions in patients for 28 days after the procedure. There were 98 patients in the study, 50 who received Hemopure and 48 who received RBC transfusions. Up to 120 g (4 units of Hemopure) could be used up to 3 days after the surgery. The use of Hemopure eliminated the need for RBC transfusions in 34% of cases, and oxygen extraction was greater in the HBOC group. This study documented that Hemopure reduced the need for allogeneic RBC transfusions without significant clinical side effects, with the exception of nonsignificant vasoconstriction reflected by increased mean blood pressure in the treatment group.[26]

A phase III, noncardiac surgery trial was initiated in 1998 in Europe and South Africa, and the goal again was to avoid RBC transfusions for 28 days after the surgery. This study enrolled 160 patients, 83 who were treated with Hemopure and 77 who were treated with RBC transfusions. Up to 210 g of Hb (7 units of Hemopure) were allowed during a 6-day treatment time. This trial obtained its goal because 43% of the patients treated with Hemopure were able to avoid RBC transfusions.

Most recently, the report of the largest clinical trial (US Phase III Orthopedic Surgery Trial, initiated in 1998) was published.[27] The ability of HBOC-201 to safely reduce or eliminate the need for perioperative transfusion was studied in orthopedic surgery patients. A randomized, single-blind, RBC-controlled, parallel-group multicenter study was conducted. Six hundred and eighty-eight patients were randomized to receive treatment with HBOC-201 (H, n = 350) or RBCs (R, n = 338) at the first transfusion decision. Primary endpoints were transfusion avoidance and blinded assessment of safety noninferiority. A total of 59.4% of patients in the H arm avoided the need for RBC transfusion. Adverse events (8.47 versus 5.88) and serious adverse events (0.35 versus 0.25) per patient were higher in the H versus R arms ($P<.001$ and $P<.01$). HBOC-201 eliminated the need for transfusion in the majority of subjects. The between-arms safety analysis (H versus R) was unfavorable and likely related to patient age, volume overload, and undertreatment, and was isolated to patients who could not be managed by using HBOC-201 alone. However, patients younger than 80 years old with moderate clinical needs may safely avoid transfusion when treated with up to 10 units of HBOC-201.

As a consequence, HBOC-2001 was approved for treatment of perioperative anemia in elective adult surgical patients in South Africa in 2001. Hemopure is approved in South Africa for the treatment of adult surgical patients who are acutely anemic, with the intention of eliminating or reducing the need for allogeneic RBC transfusions.

Per Biopure Corporation's report, Hemopure has been administered to more than eight hundred human subjects in 22 completed clinical trials, including four advanced, RBC-controlled trials in patients undergoing cardiac, vascular, general noncardiac, and orthopedic surgery, respectively. These trials represent a logical progression in the study design that has expanded the dosing limits from 4 units (120 g Hb) of

Hemopure administered after surgery over a maximum period of 3 days to 10 units (300 g Hb) administered before, during, or after surgery over a 6-day period.[28]

In the United States, phase III trials have been put on hold due to safety issues. In December 2006, the Blood Products Advisory Committee of the US Food and Drug Administration (FDA) voted against recommending that the US Navy proceed with late-phase clinical trials of Hemopure. The main reason for this was the adverse effect profile of the compound, because previous studies had shown that Hemopure could increase the risk of strokes and myocardial infarction. Hemopure's manufacturer, Biopure Corporation, is currently addressing the FDA's questions regarding the safety and efficacy of the product.

Hemopure is currently in phase III clinical trials in South Africa and Europe (**Table 5**). In the United States, Hemopure is currently under review by the FDA, and animal studies are being conducted. In March 2003, the US Naval Medical Research Center signed a collaborative research-and-development agreement with Biopure Corporation to help fund and conduct a trial on the effects of Hemopure in out-of-hospital resuscitation of patients with severe hemorrhagic shock. This trial was named Restore Effective Survival in Shock (RESUS), and more than $14 million in Congressional, Navy, Army, and Air Force funding has been given so far to support the trauma development program for Hemopure. Hemopure has also been approved for compassionate use.

PolyHeme

PolyHeme (Northfield Laboratories Inc., Evanston, Illinois) is a first-generation, pyridoxylated, polymerized Hb made from outdated human blood (**Fig. 6**). The development of PolyHeme originally began as a military project following the Vietnam War, and it has since shown great potential for both military and civilian use. It is one of the few HBOC products currently being evaluated in phase III clinical trials. It has a half-life of 24 hours, a shelf life longer than 12 months when refrigerated, and a p-50 from 28 mm to 30 mm Hg. The extraction and filtration of human Hb from RBCs is the first step in PolyHeme production. Then, using a multistep polymerization process, the purified Hb is associated into tetramers and, as the final step, is incorporated into an electrolyte solution.

Table 5 Hemopure clinical trials				
Studies (#)	Source of Patients	Hemopure Patients (n)	Control Patients (n)	Maximum Total Dose (g Hemopure)
4	Healthy volunteers	64	29	45–140
4	Nonsurgery	34	14	43–1230
3	Surgery with ANH	31	36	36–98
6	General surgery	120	70	27–245
1	Military surgery trial	26	25	300
4	Major surgery trials	531	487	120–300
22	Other clinical trials	806[a]	661	27–1230

Data do not include more than 250 postclinical trial applications in South Africa.
 Abbreviation: ANH, Acute normovolemic hemodilution.
[a] Total does not include compassionate use patients treated under emergency investigational new drug applications. *Adapted from* www.biomed.brown.edu.

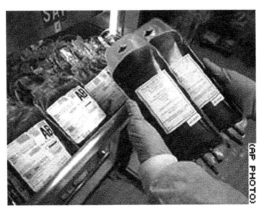

Fig. 6. MP4. (*From* www.sangart.com/hemospan/.)

PolyHeme was developed as a temporary solution to blood loss. As a military project, the focus was to develop a blood substitute to keep trauma patients alive in remote areas where allogeneic blood is not available. It is recognized that PolyHeme has a short circulation half-life of only 24 hours. Conditions requiring blood for longer than the circulation time of PolyHeme would require repeated transfusions of Poly-Heme or later replacement with donor blood. Another factor that can limit the effectiveness of PolyHeme is the fact that it is manufactured using human Hb. Although such Hb can be reclaimed from expired RBC products, it does not completely eliminate the need for donors because there must be a source of the outdated erythrocytes. The use of human Hb could limit the supply and manufacturing potential of PolyHeme.

PolyHeme: Clinical Trials

Multiple clinical trials have already been completed in the hospital setting, which have increasingly tested the safety and effectiveness of PolyHeme. Testing has included transfusion of PolyHeme during resuscitation as well as both intraoperatively and postoperatively, and has shown the effectiveness of PolyHeme at different rates, from 1 unit to 20 units. The most rapid transfusion occurred during a severe hemorrhage, in which 20 units were transfused in 20 minutes during a phase II clinical trial.

In an initial Phase II clinical trial (n = 39) up to 6 units of PolyHeme were administered in patients after acute trauma and surgery. No safety issues related to PolyHeme were reported. The plasma Hb mean was 4.8 ± 0.8 g/dL (reflecting PolyHeme Hb concentration) and RBC Hb fell to 2.9 ± 1.2 g/dL (reflecting the patients' endogenous RBC Hb), but total Hb was maintained at 7.5 ± 1.2 g/dL with infusion of 6 units (300 g) of PolyHeme.[29]

In a phase II randomized trial in 44 patients with acute trauma, PolyHeme reduced the required number of allogeneic RBC transfusions.[30] The patients (33 men, 11 women), aged from 19 to 75 years with an average Injury Severity Score of 21 ± 10, were randomized to receive RBCs (n = 23) or up to 6 units (300 g) of PolyHeme (n = 21) as their initial blood replacement after trauma and during emergent operations. There were no serious or unexpected adverse events related to PolyHeme. The PolyHeme infusion of 4.4 ± 2.0 units (mean $\pm$ standard deviation) resulted in a plasma Hb of 3.9 ± 1.3 g/dL, which accounted for 40% of the total circulating

Hb. There was no difference in total Hb between the groups before infusion (10.4 ± 2.3 g/dL control group versus 9.4 ± 1.9 g/dL experimental group). At end infusion, the experimental RBC Hb group fell to 5.8 ± 2.8 g/dL versus 10.6 ± 1.8 g/dL ($P<.05$) in the control group, although the total Hb was not different between the groups or different from that at the time of preinfusion. The total number of allogeneic RBC transfusions for the control and experimental groups was 10.4 ± 4.2 units versus 6.8 ± 3.9 units, respectively, ($P<.05$) through day 1, and 11.3 ± 4.1 units versus 7.8 ± 4.2 units, respectively, ($P = .06$) through day 3. This study documented that PolyHeme was safe in cases of acute blood loss, maintained total Hb in lieu of RBCs despite the marked fall in RBC Hb, and reduced the use of allogeneic blood. PolyHeme appeared to be a clinically useful blood substitute.

A nonrandomized, prospective trial enrolled 171 trauma or surgical patients who received rapid infusion of from 1 unit to 20 units (1,000 g, 10 L) of PolyHeme in lieu of RBCs as an initial oxygen-carrying replacement in trauma and urgent surgery.[31] The protocol simulated the unavailability of RBCs, and the progressive fall in RBC Hb in bleeding patients was quantified. The 30-day mortality of this group was compared with that of a historical control group of 300 surgical patients who refused RBCs on religious grounds. A total of 171 patients received rapid infusion of from 1 unit to 2 units (n = 45), 3 units to 4 units (n = 45), 5 units to 9 units (n = 47), and 10 units to 20 units (n = 34) of PolyHeme. Forty patients had a nadir RBC Hb≤3 g/dL (mean, 1.5 ± 0.7 g/dL), but total Hb was adequately maintained (mean, 6.8 ± 1.2 g/dL) because of plasma Hb added by PolyHeme. The 30-day mortality was 25.0% (10/40 patients) in the PolyHeme group compared with 64.5% (20/31 patients) in the historical control group at these low RBC Hb levels. Additionally, 75% of patients with RBC Hb levels less than 1 gm % survived traumatic injury after receiving PolyHeme as compared with 16% of patients in the historical control group at the same RBC Hb level. The authors concluded that Poly-Heme increases survival at life-threatening RBC Hb by maintaining total Hb (plasma and RBC Hb) in the absence of RBC transfusion. PolyHeme should be useful in the early treatment of urgent blood loss and resolve the dilemma of the unavailability of RBCs.

The USA Multicenter PolyHeme Trauma Trial was recently completed, the first trial in the United States of an HBOC in the prehospital setting using waiver of informed consent. This was a 720-patient, phase III trial in trauma patients in which subjects were randomized to receive either PolyHeme or the standard of care at the time of injury.[32] On reaching the hospital, patients in the control arm received allogeneic blood transfusion as indicated, whereas patients in the PolyHeme arm received PolyHeme for 12 hours and then received allogeneic blood as indicated. Some have commented that it was unethical to continue the study protocol for 12 hours of the in-hospital phase of the study, that is, in the absence of a requirement to administer allogeneic blood to trauma victims in the PolyHeme group upon hospital arrival.[33] Preliminary results have indicated that there was no statistically significant difference in mortality (on day 1 and day 30) between the PolyHeme and control cohorts. For detailed analyses of the results of this trial, see the article by Dr. Ernest E. Moore and colleagues elsewhere in this issue.

Hemolink

Hemolink (Hb-raffimer, Hemosol Corporation, Mississauga, Canada) is a polymerized Hb product manufactured from donated human blood and O-raffinose cross-linked to produce a polyHb. A Phase I study was performed in healthy volunteers (n = 42), of whom 33 received Hemolink, and it was well tolerated, with no evidence of organ dysfunction.[34]

Hemolink: Clinical Trials

The first phase II, randomized, controlled, single-blind, dose-escalation, multicenter trial was performed in 60 adult patients undergoing elective coronary artery bypass graft (CABG) surgery at Duke University.[35] After induction of anesthesia, autologous whole blood was collected to achieve a Hb of 7 g/dL on cardiopulmonary bypass. Patients were randomized to receive either Hemolink (treatment) or 6% hetastarch (control) in sequential, escalating dose blocks of 250 mL, 500 mL, and 750 mL. After the return of the autologous blood, allogeneic RBCs were transfused according to pre-determined Hb triggers. Serious adverse events were distributed evenly between the two groups of patients. Elevated blood pressure was more frequent in the treatment group than in the control group (16/28 mmHg versus 9/32 mmHg, P = .036). In the group of 40 patients in the 750-mL dose block, eight of the 18 treatment patients and four of the 22 control patients avoided needing allogeneic RBC transfusion (P = .093). The median volume of allogeneic RBCs transfused was lower in the treated subjects than in the control subjects (P = .042). Hemolink was well tolerated and could be effective in reducing transfusion for patients undergoing CABG surgery. Although perioperative hypertension was more frequent in the treated patients, blood pressure management prevented serious adverse sequelae.

A second phase II, dose-response study in patients receiving elective CABG surgery (n = 60) was performed in a single-blind, multicenter, placebo-controlled, open-label trial at London Health Sciences Center in Canada.[36] This study aimed to determine the dose-response of Hemolink administered in conjunction with intraoperative autologous donation in patients undergoing CABG. A secondary objective was to evaluate the effectiveness of Hemolink in reducing the incidence of the need for allogeneic RBC transfusions. Patients were randomized to receive a single dose of Hemolink or a control (10% pentastarch). Patients were sequentially enrolled in a dose block of 250 mL, 500 mL, 750 mL, and 1000 mL. Sixty patients received Hemolink (n = 30) or the control (n = 30). Hemolink was well tolerated. Most (98%) adverse events were mild or moderate in severity. There was an expected dose-dependent increase in the incidence of blood pressure increases and jaundice in Hemolink-treated patients. In a dose-pooled analysis of Hemolink versus the control, increased blood pressure (43% versus 17%), nausea (37% versus 33%), and atrial fibrillation (37% versus 17%) were the most frequently reported adverse events. All serious adverse events were considered unrelated or unlikely to be related to the study drug. No Hemolink-treated patient required an intraoperative allogeneic RBC transfusion, compared with 5 (17%) pentastarch-treated patients (P = .052). This advantage of Hemolink was maintained at 24 hours after surgery (7% versus 37%; P = .010) and up to 5 days after surgery (10% versus 47%; P = .0034). Hemolink was effective in facilitating decreased exposure or avoidance of allogeneic RBC transfusions when used in conjunction with intraoperative autologous donation.

A phase III, multicenter clinical trial was undertaken next. The purpose of this study was to determine if intraoperative autologous donation alone or in conjunction with Hemolink confers a reduction in RBC or blood component transfusion compared with results in standard clinical practice. The trial was a multicenter, randomized, double-blind study to determine the efficacy and safety of Hemolink versus 10% pentastarch when used to facilitate intraoperative autologous donation in 299 patients undergoing primary CABG. The patients received Hemolink or pentastarch as an adjunct to intraoperative autologous donation immediately before cardiopulmonary bypass. Results were compared with transfusion requirements for 150 matched patients in the reference group. The frequency of allogeneic RBC transfusion in the Hemolink, pentastarch, and reference groups was 56%, 76%, and 95%, respectively. The number of allogeneic RBC units used was 49 in the Hemolink group, 104 in the pentastarch group, and 480 in the reference group ($P<.001$). The total number of non-RBC units administered was 150 in the Hemolink group, 238 in the pentastarch group, and 270 in the reference group. In this study, patients treated with Hemolink in conjunction with intraoperative autologous donation received fewer transfusions overall and a lower volume of allogeneic RBCs and non-RBC allogeneic blood products than did those in the two comparison groups. This potentially confers a real benefit on the overall blood supply by decreasing use and increasing availability.

In light of the limited resources available to Hemosol Corporation, as well as the time and expense likely required to address certain adverse results noted in the course of the clinical trials of Hemolink, the company elected to discontinue further development of Hemolink in June 2004.

Maleimide PEG-Hb

Maleimide PEG-Hb (MP4) (Sangart Inc., San Diego, California) is a polyethylene glycol–conjugated human Hb currently undergoing clinical trials in Europe as a colloid oxygen therapeutic and not as a blood substitute.[37] To further increase the circulation time, Hb can be linked to a macromolecule to increase its size. Human or bovine Hb that is conjugated with polyethylene glycol (PEG) is protected from renal excretion. The PEG-Hb has a larger molecular size and has a viscosity lower than whole blood but higher than colloids in clinical use.

MP4 was developed by introducing additional surface thiols with iminothiolane onto the Hb. This process usually adds about six additional thiols, and it is then linked to on average eight PEG-5000. MP4 then requires no more purification steps. MP4 has a lower Hb concentration, higher viscosity (but lower than blood), higher oxygen-affinity, and higher colloidal oncotic pressure than most other HBOCs in development (**Table 6**). MP4 did demonstrate an improvement in microcirculatory blood flow and tissue oxygenation in animal studies. In animal models, MP4 has been shown to be effective in reversing lactic acidosis in studies of hemorrhagic shock.[38] Adverse effects associated with the vasoactive properties of first-generation blood substitutes are not seen with MP4. At relatively low concentrations, MP4 is capable of transporting

Table 6
Characteristics of HBOCs

Characteristics	Product (Company)		
	PolyHeme (Northfield Laboratories Inc.)	Hemopure (Biopure Corporation)	MP4 (Sangart Inc.)
Volume (ml)	500	250	250
Hb concentration (g/dl)	10	13	4.3
Hb mass (g)	50	~30	~10
P_{50} (mm Hg)	26–32	38	5
Methemoglobin (%)	<8.0	<15.0	<10.0
Tetramer (%)	≤1.0	≤3.0	<1.0
Shelf life (years)	>1	3	>1

large amounts of oxygen. Pharmacokinetic analysis of plasma Hb yielded an estimated half-life of 43 hours in subjects in the phase I trial who received 100 mg/kg.

MP4: Clinical Trials

Sangart Inc. announced positive results from a phase I study of MP4 in 2005.[39] A Phase Ib/II clinical trial evaluated increasing doses of MP4 in orthopedic surgery patients (n = 30), with doses of from 200 mL to 1000 mL of either MP4 or Ringer's acetate before induction of spinal anesthesia was subsequently completed. This study demonstrated that MP4 was well tolerated at these doses, with no new safety concerns raised.[40]

A Phase II trial, conducted in Sweden, involved 90 patients undergoing hip arthroplasty in a multicenter, double-blind, clinical trial. Patients were randomized to receive either MP4 or Ringer's acetate (control) before induction of spinal anesthesia. MP4 was found to be well tolerated in the study group, with no serious adverse effects attributed to the product during the trial period. The percentage of hypotensive episodes in the MP4 group was about 45%, compared with 87% among those in the control group. Incidence of intraoperative vasopressor use was about 15% in the MP4 group, compared with 32% among those in the control group. A special feature of this study was Holter monitoring, starting 1 hour before induction of anesthesia and continued for 24 hours. Blinded analysis of these data did not find any significant imbalances or safety concerns.[41]

A single-center, double-blind, phase II study of MP4 was completed in November 2007 at the Johns Hopkins Medical Center in Baltimore. In this study, patients undergoing elective open prostatectomy were randomly assigned to receive either crystalloid (Ringer's solution) or MP4 after an estimated surgical blood loss of 250 mL. A special feature of this study was the assessment of pulmonary artery hemodynamics using transesophageal echo (ClinicalTrials.gov Identifier NCT00425334).

A randomized, single-blind, controlled, phase II pilot study of the use of MP4 compared with colloid (Voluven, Fresenius Kabi, BAD Homburg, Germany [6% hydroxyethyl starch 130/0.4 in 0.9% sodium chloride], a commercial starch-based plasma expander) to evaluate vascular resistance and blood flow in the forearm and to assess local skin blood flow and tissue oxygenation in an ischemic region of the foot in patients with chronic critical limb ischemia recently completed at the Karolinska University Hospital in Stockholm, Sweden. The main study objective was to investigate the effect of MP4 on vascular resistance and demonstrate the absence of vasoconstriction in patients with chronic critical limb ischemia. The secondary study objective was to evaluate the effects of MP4 on local skin blood flow and tissue oxygenation in an ischemic region of the foot in these patients.

MP4 is undergoing further evaluation in two pivotal, multicenter, international, double-blind, controlled, phase III studies in Europe. One study (a prevention trial) completed enrollment of 376 patients at 18 centers in six countries in May 2008 and evaluated the ability of MP4 to prevent acute hypotension in orthopedic surgery patients undergoing first-time hip replacement procedures under spinal anesthesia. The primary objective was to demonstrate that MP4 is a superior colloid compared with Voluven for preventing hypotensive episodes during the operative and early postoperative period. The secondary objective was to show that MP4 can also reduce the incidence of operative and postoperative morbidity. (Additional details can be found at http://clinicaltrials.gov/NCT00420277).

An additional study (a treatment trial) completed enrollment of 474 patients at 21 centers in five countries in March 2008 and evaluated the ability of MP4 to treat acute hypotension in orthopedic surgery patients undergoing first-time hip replacement procedures under spinal anesthesia. The primary objective was to demonstrate that MP4 is a superior colloid compared with Voluven for treating hypotensive episodes during the operative period. The secondary objective was to show that MP4 can also reduce the incidence of operative and postoperative morbidity. (Additional details can be found at http://clinicaltrials.gov/ct/show/NCT00420277?order=1).

RECOMBINANT HUMAN HEMOGLOBIN

Recombinant human Hb (rHb) is manufactured using *Escherichia coli* with recombinant technology. This technology can be used to induce a variety of cell types to synthesize functional Hb. In addition, modifications of the Hb molecular structure can alter the properties of the molecule, allowing researchers to create Hbs with improved functionality or enhanced safety when used as Hb therapeutics. One very positive feature of rHb is that it can be manufactured resulting in an unlimited supply.

Two first-generation HBOCs were under development by Baxter Hemoglobin Therapeutics and Somatogen (Boulder, Colorado) during the 1990s, DCIHb (HemAssist) and a modified rHb (rHb1.1, Optro), respectively. Each of these products had circumvented the safety concerns arising from dimerization of the Hb tetramer by cross-linking the alpha chains (either chemically in the case of DCIHb or through recombinant engineering with rHb1.1).[42]

rHb1.1 was a first-generation HBOC with a nitric oxide scavenging rate similar to that of native human Hb. rHb2.0 was a second-generation HBOC, created via genetic manipulation of the distal heme pocket of both the alpha and beta subunits of Hb, leading to steric hindrance for nitric oxide entry, with a nitric oxide scavenging rate from 20- to 30-fold lower than rHb1.1 but with maintenance of effective oxygen binding and release.[43] Preclinical animal studies were promising. rHb2.0 was associated with decreased pulmonary hypertension, diminished capacity to scavenge nitric oxide, and lack of modulation of pulmonary vascular permeability. These findings therefore lend promise for the use of HBOCs with low nitric oxide reactivity as oxygen therapeutics.

rHb2.0 has been investigated in a swine model of uncontrolled hemorrhage. rHb2.0 performed as well as heterologous blood for resuscitation in hemorrhage, did not cause sustained pulmonary hypertension, maintained adequate cardiac output and oxygen delivery, and was superior to lactated Ringer's solution and the first-generation HBOC DCIHb in survival rates.[44] Additional preclinical studies documented positive results.[45–48] Although rHb2.0 appeared promising, no clinical trials were performed and Baxter Corporation suspended funding of this initiative.

NEXT-GENERATION HBOCs

A number of new, advanced HBOCs are undergoing development.[49] A complete discussion of these HBOCs is beyond the scope of this review. A few interesting compounds deserve mention.

Pyridoxylated Hb polyoxyethylene conjugate (PHP, Apex Bioscience, Chapel Hill, North Carolina) is a conjugated Hb that is currently undergoing a phase III trial in patients with shock associated with systemic inflammatory response syndrome. The study has been designed to evaluate the safety and efficacy of continuous intravenous infusion of PHP plus conventional vasopressor treatment versus continuous intravenous infusion of Plasma-lyte A (Baxter Healthcare Corp., Deerfield, Illinois) plus conventional vasopressors as a treatment for restoring hemodynamic stability in patients with systemic inflammatory response syndrome with shock. The trial has an estimated enrollment of 1000 patients, and the study start date was March 2001 (ClinicalTrials.gov Identifier NCT00021502).

For HBOCs cross-linked with enzymes, there has been an effort to synthesize compounds that not only perform the function of carrying oxygen, as do the molecules mentioned previously, but also harbor some of the enzyme activity that normal RBCs possess. PolyHb has been cross-linked with catalase and superoxide dismutase to form a compound that, in animal models, can not only carry oxygen but also remove oxygen radicals that are responsible for ischemia reperfusion injuries (**Figs. 7** and **8**).[50] PolyHb has also been cross-linked with tyrosinase to form a soluble complex that can carry oxygen and decrease the systemic levels of tyrosine. This agent can help increase the efficacy of chemotherapy and radiation therapy in tumor tissue, and in a melanoma model, it has been shown to delay tumor growth without having significant adverse effects.

Cellular HBOCs

Cellular HBOCs consist of Hb molecules encapsulated inside oxygen carriers of different natures, aimed at mimicking features of RBCs. The advantages of cellular HBOCs consist of protecting the surrounding tissues and blood components from direct contact with potentially toxic tetrameric Hb, avoiding the Hb colloidal osmotic effect, prolonging Hb circulation half-life, and not requiring the direct modification of the Hb molecule. Additionally, with the application of nanotechnology, it is possible to achieve a submicron-sized oxygen carrier and thus ensure oxygen availability to all body compartments. Two types of cellular HBOCs have been studied: liposome systems and polymeric micro/nanoparticle systems.[51]

Efforts have been made to encapsulate Hb within a lipid membrane to create a compound capable of carrying oxygen while not being associated with significant

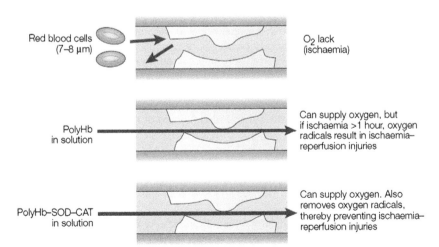

Fig. 7. In conditions of tissue ischemia, RBCs may not be able to get to the location of the ischemia due to their size. PolyHb can get there but will provide oxygen for only a short period. PolyHb cross-linked with superoxide dismutase (SOD) and catalase (CAT) can supply oxygen and remove oxygen radicals, thus treating ischemic-reperfusion injury. (*From* Chang TMS. Therapeutic applications of polymeric artificial cells. Nature Reviews 2005;4:221–35; with permission.)

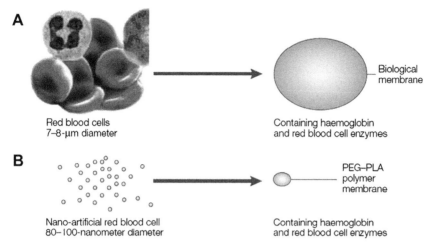

Fig. 8. (A, B) RBCs can circulate freely to carry out their functions. Polymeric artificial RBCs can be prepared, but they have to be nanodimensional and with special membrane materials (for example, polyethylene glycol–polylactide (PEG–PLA) copolymer) for them to circulate freely. (*From* Chang TMS. Therapeutic applications of polymeric artificial cells. Nature Reviews 2005;4:221–35; with permission.)

vasoconstriction. These liposomes appear to be retained in plasma for a significant period. However, they are difficult to produce and can activate the reticuloendothelial system, the complement pathway, and platelets. At present, the only institutions working actively on this product are in Japan.

The ultimate RBC substitute would contain not only Hb but also other contents of the RBC encapsulated in an artificial membrane. However, production of such a product would be extremely challenging. Efforts have been made to use polyactide, a biodegradable polymer that is converted to lactic acid in the body, to create artificial RBCs. These cells contain Hb along with the RBC enzyme complement, including superoxide dismutase, methemoglobin reductase, and catalase. (For more on this topic, see the article by Chang elsewhere in this issue.)

Modifying the method of preparing microdimensional, polymeric, artificial cells can result in the creation of nanodimensional artificial cells. In the case of blood substitutes, nanodimensional liposomes of about 200 nm that contain Hb have been prepared. Biodegradable polymer membranes are being used to form nanodimensional, artificial RBCs as a third-generation blood substitute. These nanodimensional, artificial RBCs (80–150 nm in diameter) contain all the RBC enzymes. Recent studies show that using a polyethylene glycol–polylactide (PEG-PLA) copolymer membrane, it is possible to increase the circulation time of these nanodimensional, artificial RBCs to double that of polyHb.

ADVERSE EFFECTS OF HBOCs

Adverse effects associated with HBOCs include hypertension, abdominal pain, skin rash, diarrhea, jaundice, hemoglobinuria, oliguria, fever, stroke, and laboratory anomalies such as an elevation in lipase levels. Although most of these side effects were transient and clinically asymptomatic, many clinical trials involving these agents have been discontinued or held due to the associated adverse side effects. Although current formulations appear to cause fewer and less severe side effects compared with previous products, there remain concerns associated with HBOCs, including the following:

Vasoactivity—HBOC products are known to cause vasoconstrictive effects. As nitric oxide binds to Hb, nitric oxide becomes less available to cause vascular smooth muscle relaxation. Hence, vasoconstricition occurs.

Hemostasis—Studies have shown an increased hemostatic effect in HBOCs due to reversal of the inhibition effect of nitric oxide on platelet aggregation.

Gastrointestinal side effects—Studies have observed gastrointestinal side effects such as nausea, vomiting, diarrhea, and bloating. The binding of nitrous oxide to gastrointestinal intestine tissues is the proposed cause.

Interference with laboratory assays—High concentrations of Hb in plasma due to the infusion of HBOCs interfere with laboratory assays. Tests for liver enzymes, bilirubin, amylase, and other substances often yield inaccurate results because of the presence of HBOCs.

It has been difficult to discern whether the adverse events that have been observed following the infusion of HBOCs in patients subjected to elective orthopedic procedures, cardiopulmonary bypass surgery, and vascular surgical procedures are related solely to the HBOCs or to other treatments administered to these patients during their routine care. Along with all three of the HBOCs, the patients received Ringer's d,l-lactate as the resuscitative fluid, Ringer's d,l-lactate in the excipient medium for the HBOC, and liquid preserved red blood cells that had been stored at 4°C for longer than 2 weeks. The Ringer's d,l-lactate solution has been shown to be toxic in both animals and patients. The current formulation of Ringer's lactate contains only the l-isomer which has been shown in animals to be less toxic than the d-isomer of lactate. In a recent publication morbidity and mortality have been reported associated with the length of storage of red blood cells at 4°C in patients subjected to reoperative cardiac surgery. Current clinical studies to assess the safety and therapeutic effectiveness of a HBOC must consider the effects of the composition of the resuscitation solution (Ringer's l-lactate), the composition of the excipient medium (Ringer's l-lactate or 0.9% NaCl) for the HBOC, and the length of storage of the liquid preserved red blood cells infused with the HBOC.[52]

A recent meta-analysis reviewed data on death and myocardial infarction as outcome variables in 16 trials in adult patients (n = 3711) involving five different HBOCs in varied patient populations.[53] They reported a statistically significant increase in the risk of death (164 versus 123 deaths; relative risk [RR] 1.30, 95% CI, 1.05–1.61) and the risk of myocardial infarction (59 versus 16 myocardial infarctions; RR 2.71; 95% CI, 1.67–4.40). There are, however, many limitations to this analysis.[54] For instance, multiple products (HemAssist, PolyHeme, Hemolink, Hemopure, MP4) were all included in this analysis, and there was a lack of consistent monitoring of cardiac events in these studies, a lack of consistent treatment in the perioperative period to prevent cardiac events in the surgical studies, no identification of specific cardiac risk in patients enrolled in these studies, and a lack of control for risk of myocardial events and mortality that may have been related to allogeneic transfusion.[55,56]

But these adverse effects of HBOCs may also occur with the transfusion of aged human RBCs. It has been documented that as human blood is stored, hemolysis occurs and increased concentrations of free Hb are present in these units of blood.[57] Abnormal hemolysis in an individual RBC unit may be caused by several factors, including inappropriate handling during the processing of blood, inappropriate or extended duration of storage, bacterial hemolysins, antibodies that cause complement lysis, defects in the RBC membrane, or an abnormality in the blood donor. The acceptable level of hemolysis has not been established in North America, but the value of 1% is currently used to assess biocompatibility of blood storage materials.[58]

Free plasma Hb, in addition to generating reactive oxygen species such as the hydroxyl and superoxide radicals, is also a potent scavenger of nitric oxide. Nitric oxide, which is normally produced by the endothelium, regulates basal vasodilator tone, inhibits platelet and hemostatic activation, and reduces superoxide levels through radical–radical scavenging. The vasodilator activity of nitric oxide is possible only because most Hb is normally compartmentalized within erythrocytes.

The clinical consequences of RBC storage for patients who are critically ill are particularly concerning.[59] Duration of RBC storage has been associated with adverse outcomes. In patients undergoing cardiac surgery, transfusion of RBCs that had been stored for more than 2 weeks was associated with a significantly increased risk of postoperative complications as well as reduced short-term and long-term survival.[60] Additional studies have documented significant risks associated with RBC transfusion[61–63] and lack of efficacy.[64,65]

SUMMARY

There is still a significant unmet medical need for HBOCs in a variety of medical situations. There are now available additional viable approaches to modify the intrinsic biologic properties of Hb to produce improved HBOCs. The ultimate goal is availability of an HBOC for clinical use in appropriate clinical situations.

Polymerized Hb preparations have proved most successful in clinical trials due to their improved side effect profile. The goal is to evaluate blood substitutes with enhanced intravascular retention, reduced osmotic activity, and attenuated hemodynamic derangements such as vasoconstriction. Although not without substantial morbidity and mortality, the current safety of allogeneic blood transfusion demands that comparative studies show minimal adverse effects as well as efficacy and potential for novel applications.

REFERENCES

1. Winslow RM. Current status of oxygen carriers ("blood substitutes"): 2006. Vox Sang 2006;91(2):102–10.
2. Habler O, Pape A, Meier J, et al. Artificial oxygen carriers as an alternative to red blood cell transfusion. Anaesthesist 2005;54(8):741–54.
3. Ness PM, Cushing MM. Oxygen therapeutics: pursuit of an alternative to the donor red blood cell. Arch Pathol Lab Med 2007;131:734–41.
4. Sullivan MT, Cotten R, Read EJ, et al. Blood collection and transfusion in the United States in 2001. Transfusion 2007;47:385–94.
5. Zou S, Musavi F, Notari EP 4th, et al. ARCNET Research Group. Changing age distribution of the blood donor population in the United States. Transfusion 2008;48(2):251–7.
6. Spiess BD. Risks of transfusions: outcome focus. Transfusion 2004;4:4S–14S.
7. Sazama K. The ethics of blood management. Vox Sang 2007;92:95–102.
8. Cable R, Carlson B, Chambers L, et al. Practice guidelines for blood transfusion: a compilation from recent peer-reviewed literature. Washington, DC: American National Red Cross; 2002.
9. Available at: www.hemopure.com. Accessed November 23, 2008.

10. Tsai AG, Cabrales P, Intaglietta M. Oxygen-carrying blood substitutes: a microvascular perspective. Expert Opin Biol Ther 2004;4(7):1147–57.

11. Stowell CP, Levin J, Speiss BD, et al. Progress in the development of RBC substitutes. Transfusion 2001;41:287–99.

12. Goodnough LT, Brecher ME, Kanter MH, et al. Transfusion medicine: first of two parts. N Engl J Med 1999;340:438–47.

13. Winslow RM. Vasoconstriction and the efficacy of hemoglobin-based blood substitutes. Transfus Clin Biol 1994;1(1):9–14.

14. Standl T. Haemoglobin-based erythrocyte transfusion substitutes. Expert Opin Biol Ther 2001;1(5):831–43.

15. Stowell CP. What happened to blood substitutes? Transfus Clin Biol 2005;12:374–9.

16. Estep T, Bucci E, Farmer M, et al. Basic science focus on blood substitutes: a summary of the NHLBI Division of Blood Diseases and Resources Working Group Workshop, March 1, 2006. Transfusion 2008;48:776–82.

17. Meisner FG, Kemming GI, Habler OP, et al. Diaspirin crosslinked hemoglobin enables extreme hemodilution beyond the critical hematocrit. Crit Care Med 2001;29(4):829–38.

18. Saxena R, Wihnhoud AD, Carton H, et al. Controlled safety study of a hemoglobin-based oxygen carrier, DCLHb, in acute ischemic stroke. Stroke 1999;30:993–6.

19. Sloan EP, Koenigsberg M, Gens D, et al. Diaspirin cross-linked hemoglobin (DCLHb) in the treatment of severe traumatic hemorrhagic shock: a randomized controlled efficacy trial. JAMA 1999;282:1857–64.

20. Schubert A, Przybelski RJ, Eidt JF, et al. Perioperative Avoidance or Reduction of Transfusion Trial (PARTT) Study Group. Diaspirin-crosslinked hemoglobin reduces blood transfusion in noncardiac surgery: a multicenter, randomized, controlled, double-blinded trial. Anesth Analg 2003;97(2):323–32.

21. Lamy ML, Daily EK, Brichant JF, et al. Randomized trial of diaspirin cross-linked hemoglobin solution as an alternative to blood transfusion after cardiac surgery. The DCLHb Cardiac Surgery Trial Collaborative Group. Anesthesiology 2000;92(3):646–56.

22. Schubert A, O'Hara JF Jr, Przybelski RJ, et al. Effect of diaspirin crosslinked hemoglobin (DCLHb HemAssist) during high blood loss surgery on selected indices of organ function. Artif Cells Blood Substit Immobil Biotechnol 2002;30(4):259–83.

23. Cabrales P, Tsai AG, Intaglietta M. Balance between vasoconstriction and enhanced oxygen delivery. Transfusion 2008;48(10):2087–95.

24. LaMuraglia GM, O'Hara PJ, Baker WH, et al. The reduction of allogeneic transfusion requirements in aortic surgery with a hemoglobin-based solution. J Vasc Surg 2000;31(2):299–308.

25. Sprung J, Kindscher JD, Wahr JA, et al. The use of bovine hemoglobin glutamer-250 (Hemopure) in surgical patients: results of a multicenter, randomized, single-blinded trial. Anesth Analg 2002;94(4):799–808.

26. Levy JH, Goodnough LT, Greilich PE, et al. Polymerized bovine hemoglobin solution as a replacement for allogeneic red blood cell transfusion after cardiac surgery: results of a randomized, double-blind trial. J Thorac Cardiovasc Surg 2002;124:35–42.

27. Jahr JS, MacKenzie C, Pearce LB, et al. HBOC-201 as an alternative to blood transfusion: efficacy and safety evaluation in a multicenter phase III trial in elective orthopedic surgery. J Trauma 2008;64(6):1484–97.
28. Jahr JS, Moallempour M, Lim JC. HBOC-201, hemoglobin glutamer-250 (bovine), Hemopure (Biopure Corporation). Expert Opin Biol Ther 2008;8(9):1425–33.
29. Gould SA, Moore EE, Moore FA, et al. Clinical utility of human polymerized hemoglobin as a blood substitute after acute trauma and urgent surgery. J Trauma 1997;43(2):325–31 [discussion: 331–2].
30. Gould SA, Moore EE, Hoyt DB, et al. The first randomized trial of human polymerized hemoglobin as a blood substitute in acute trauma and emergent surgery. J Am Coll Surg 1998;187(2):113–20 [discussion: 120–2].
31. Gould SA, Moore EE, Hoyt DB, et al. The life-sustaining capacity of human polymerized hemoglobin when red cells might be unavailable. J Am Coll Surg 2002; 195(4):445–52 [discussion: 452–5].
32. Moore EE, Moore FA, Fabian TC, et al. Human polymerized hemoglobin for the treatment of hemorrhagic shock when blood is unavailable: the USA Multicenter Trial. J Am Coll Surg, in press.
33. Apte SS. Blood substitutes—the polyheme trials. Crossroads: where medicine and the humanities meet. Mcgill J Med 2008;11(1):59–65.
34. Carmichael FJ, Ali AC, Campbell JA, et al. A phase I study of oxidized raffinose cross-linked human hemoglobin. Crit Care Med 2000;28(7):2283–92.
35. Hill SE, Gottschalk LI, Grichnik K. Safety and preliminary efficacy of hemoglobin raffimer for patients undergoing coronary artery bypass surgery. J Cardiothorac Vasc Anesth 2002;16(6):695–702.
36. Cheng DC, Mazer CD, Martineau R, et al. A phase II dose-response study of hemoglobin raffimer (Hemolink) in elective coronary artery bypass surgery. J Thorac Cardiovasc Surg 2004;127(1):79–86.
37. Vandegriff KD, Malavalli A, Wooldridge J, et al. MP4, a new nonvasoactive PEG-Hb conjugate. Transfusion 2003;43(4):509–16.
38. Young MA, Riddez L, Kjellström BT, et al. MalPEG-hemoglobin (MP4) improves hemodynamics, acid-base status, and survival after uncontrolled hemorrhage in anesthetized swine. Crit Care Med 2005;33(8):1794–804.
39. Bjorkholm M, Fagrell B, Przybelski R, et al. A phase I single blind clinical trial of a new oxygen transport agent (MP4), human hemoglobin modified with maleimide-activated polyethylene glycol. Haematologica 2005;90:505–15.
40. Olofsson C, Nygårds EB, Ponzer S, et al. A randomized, single-blind, increasing dose safety trial of an oxygen-carrying plasma expander (Hemospan) administered to orthopedic surgery patients with spinal anesthesia. Transfus Med 2008;18:28–39.
41. Olofsson N, Ahl T, Johansson T, et al. A multicenter clinical study of the safety and activity of maleimide-polyethylene glycol hemoglobin (Hemospan) in patients undergoing major orthopedic surgery. Anesthesiology 2006;105:1153–63.
42. Burhop KE. The development of a second-generation, designer, recombinant hemoglobin. In: Kobayashi K, Tsuchida E, Horinouchi H, editors. Artificial Oxygen Carrier, Keio University International Symposia for Life Sciences and Medicine, vol. 12. Tokyo: Springer's; 2005. p. 127–35.
43. Resta TC, Walker BR, Eichinger M, et al. Rate of NO scavenging alters effects of recombinant hemoglobin solutions on pulmonary vasoreactivity. J Appl Physiol 2002;93:1327–36.

44. Malhotra AK, Kelly ME, Miller PR, et al. Resuscitation with a novel hemoglobin-based oxygen carrier in a swine model of uncontrolled perioperative hemorrhage. J Trauma 2003;54(5):915–24.
45. Fronticelli C, Koehler RC, Brinigar WS. Recombinant hemoglobins as artificial oxygen carriers. Artif Cells Blood Substit Immobil Biotechnol 2007;35: 45–52.
46. Hermann J, Corso C, Messmer KF. Resuscitation with recombinant hemoglobin rHb2.0 in a rodent model of hemorrhagic shock. Anesthesiology 2007;107(2): 273–80.
47. Raat NJ, Liu J, Doyle MP, et al. Effects of recombinant hemoglobin solutions rHb2.0 and rHb1.1 on blood pressure, intestinal blood flow, and gut oxygenation in a rat model of hemorrhagic shock. J Lab Clin Med 2005;145(1):21–32.
48. Von Dobschuetz E, Hutter J, Hoffmann T, et al. Recombinant human hemoglobin with reduced nitric oxide scavenging capacity restores effectively pancreatic microcirculatory disorders in hemorrhagic shock. Anesthesiology 2004;100(6): 1484–90.
49. Kim HW, Greenburg AG. Toward 21st century blood component replacement therapeutics: artificial oxygen carriers, platelet substitutes, recombinant clotting factors, and others. Artif Cells Blood Substit Immobil Biotechnol 2006;34: 537–50.
50. Chang TM. Blood substitutes based on nanobiotechnology. Trends Biotechnol 2006;24(8):372–7.
51. Piras AM, Dessy A, Chiellini F, et al. Polymeric nanoparticles for hemoglobin-based oxygen carriers. Biochim Biophys Acta 2008;1784(10):1454–61.
52. Valeri CR, Ragno G, Veech RL. Severe adverse events associated with hemoglobin based oxygen carriers: role of resuscitative fluids and liquid preserved RBC. Transfus Apher Sci 2008;39:205–11.
53. Natanson C, Kern SJ, Lurie P, et al. Cell-free hemoglobin-based blood substitutes and risk of myocardial infarction and death. JAMA 2008;299(19):2304–12.
54. Fergusson DA, McIntyre L. The future of clinical trials evaluating blood substitutes [editorial]. JAMA 2008;299:2324–46.
55. Rao SV, Jollis JG, Harrington RA, et al. Relationship of blood transfusion and clinical outcomes in patients with acute coronary syndromes. JAMA 2004;292(13): 1555–62.
56. Gerber DR. Transfusion of packed red blood cells in patients with ischemic heart disease. Crit Care Med 2008;36(4):1068–74.
57. Gammon RR, Strayer SA, Avery NL, et al. Hemolysis during leukocyte-reduction filtration of stored red blood cells. Ann Clin Lab Sci 2000;30(2):195–9.
58. Sowemimo-Coker SO. Red blood cell hemolysis during processing. Transfus Med Rev 2002;16(1):46–60.
59. Tinmouth A, Fergusson D, Yee IC, et al. ABLE Investigators; Canadian Critical Care Trials Group. Clinical consequences of red cell storage in the critically ill. Transfusion 2006;46(11):2014–27.
60. Koch CG, Li L, Sessler DI, et al. Duration of red cell storage and complications after cardiac surgery. N Engl J Med 2008;358(12):1229–39.
61. Napolitano LM. Cumulative risks of early red blood cell transfusion. J Trauma 2006;60(Suppl 6):S26–34.
62. Malone DL, Dunne J, Tracy JK, et al. Blood transfusion, independent of shock severity, is associated with worse outcome in trauma. J Trauma 2003;54(5): 898–905.

63. Dunne JR, Malone DL, Tracy JK, et al. Allogeneic blood transfusion in the first 24 hours after trauma is associated with increased SIRS and death. Surg Infect (Larchmt) 2004;5(4):395–404.
64. Napolitano LM, Corwin HL. Efficacy of blood transfusion in the critically ill. Crit Care Clin 2004;20(2):255–8, Review.
65. Marik PE, Corwin HL. Efficacy of red blood cell transfusion in the critically ill: a systematic review of the literature. Crit Care Med 2008;36(9):2667–74.

Comparison of Hemoglobin-based Oxygen Carriers to Stored Human Red Blood Cells

Alexander L. Eastman, MD[a], Joseph P. Minei, MD[a,b],*

KEYWORDS

- Hemoglobin based oxygen carrier • Transfusion
- Packed red blood cells • Alternatives to transfusion
- Military transfusion

Since the inception of allogeneic blood transfusion (ABT), the search for an alternative to the use of stored packed red blood cells (PRBCs) has been underway. Because of several problems with the transfusion of stored red blood cells (RBCs), several alternatives to PRBC transfusion have been researched and advocated.[1,2] Most recently, particularly over the last 10 years, modified hemoglobin solutions in the form of hemoglobin-based oxygen carriers (HBOCs) have made significant strides toward becoming clinically available and useful.[3]

A number of recent review articles have documented progress in the development of HBOCs as a useful clinical alternative.[4] In addition to these articles, other investigators have attempted to elucidate the optimal characteristics of a substitute for the transfusion of stored PRBCs (**Box 1**).[5,6] Many of these characteristics have made the list in a direct attempt to counter one or more of the deleterious effects of transfusion of stored PRBCs; however, continued questions regarding the safety of these products have kept them from full Food and Drug Administration approval and from widespread implementation into clinical practice.

To understand the controversies and the search for an optimal blood substitute, one must evaluate the characteristics of the present HBOCs in detail, examine the

[a] Department of Surgery, Division of Burn, Trauma and Critical Care, University of Texas Southwestern Medical Center, 5323 Harry Hines Blvd., Dallas, TX 75390-9158, USA
[b] Parkland Memorial Hospital, 5201 Harry Hines Boulevard, Dallas, TX 75235, USA
* Corresponding author. Department of Surgery/BTCC E5.508, UT Southwestern, 5323 Harry Hines Blvd., Dallas, TX 75390-9158.
E-mail address: joseph.minei@utsouthwestern.edu (J.P. Minei).

Crit Care Clin 25 (2009) 303–310
doi:10.1016/j.ccc.2008.12.009
0749-0704/08/$ – see front matter © 2009 Elsevier Inc. All rights reserved.
criticalcare.theclinics.com

Box 1
Characteristics of an optimal packed red blood cell substitute

Similar to natural hemoglobin

    Oxygen delivery

    CO_2 transport

Nonreactive/nonantigenic

Immediately available

Easy to administer

Stable at room temperature/long-term storage

Nonoxidative/No free radical formation

Data from Jahr JS, Walker V, Monoocheri K, et al. Blood substitutes as pharmacotherapies in clinical practice. Curr Opin Anaesthesiol 2007;20(4):325–30.

---

deleterious effects of the administration of stored PRBCs, and then by comparing the two, attempt to find some alternative strategies.

CHARACTERISTICS OF HEMOGLOBIN-BASED OXYGEN CARRIERS

Many advances in exogenous hemoglobin administration have occurred since the original use of stroma-free hemoglobin in the 1970s. Today, two principal products have garnered most of the clinical attention and appear to be poised to make the first significant clinical impact. PolyHeme (Northfield Laboratories, Inc., Evanston, Illinois) and Hemopure (HBOC-201; Biopure Corporation, Cambridge, Massachusetts) have been tested in phase III clinical trials and represent the present potential for HBOC usage. **Table 1** lists some of the basic characteristics of these two HBOCs.

PolyHeme is made from purified human hemoglobin extracted from human RBCs and is processed to make a polymerized product free of impurities and potential infectious agents. Like HBOC-201, because it is devoid of cellular components, PolyHeme is completely nonantigenic and therefore requires no cross-matching or typing before transfusion. One unit of PolyHeme contains approximately 50 g of hemoglobin, similar to that contained in a single unit of PRBCs. PolyHeme requires refrigerated storage,

Table 1
Characteristics of hemoglobin-based oxygen carriers and stored packed red blood cells

	PRBCs	HBOC-201	PolyHeme
Source	Human	Bovine	Human
Hemoglobin (g/dL)	13	13	10
Average molecular weight (kd)	—	250	150
P_{50}	26	43	28–30
pH	6.8–7.1	7.6–7.9	unknown
Osmolarity	—	290–310	unknown

Adapted from Jahr JS, Walker V, Monoocheri K, et al. Blood substitutes as pharmacotherapies in clinical practice. Curr Opin Anaesthesiol 2007;20(4):325–30; with permission.

whereas HBOC-201 can be stored at room temperature. PolyHeme and HBOC-201 are transportable in volumes significantly smaller than a unit of PRBCs.

To date, PolyHeme has been extensively studied in trauma or emergency surgery patients who have massive hemorrhage. In the initial, sentinel study of HBOCs to date in this population, 171 patients received one to 20 units of PolyHeme. Forty (23.4%) of these patients had a significant drop in measured RBC hemoglobin (<3 g/dL); however, total hemoglobin was maintained by the addition of PolyHeme. The investigators observed a mortality rate of 25%, which compared favorably to a rate of 64% in matched historical control subjects who had similar hemoglobin levels.[7] This enthusiasm was somewhat tempered when Northfield Laboratories released preliminary data from a much larger, phase III trial of PolyHeme. In this multicenter trial of 25 trauma centers in the United States, 13.2% of patients receiving PolyHeme died compared with 9.6% of patients in the control group. In fact, controversy over the "waiver of informed consent" status of this study has injected delays into the prehospital study of other HBOC products.

Hemopure, or HBOC-201, is composed of glutaraldehyde cross-linked bovine hemoglobin in a modified lactated Ringer's solution. It is an oxygen-carrying solution that increases plasma and total hemoglobin concentrations. There are two potential mechanisms by which HBOC-201 enhances oxygen transport. By promoting convective and diffusive oxygen delivery, HBOC-201 administration results in an increase in oxygen delivery (1) secondary to an increased oxygen-carrying capacity of the plasma, and (2) through changes in the rheology of the blood itself. By virtue of its viscosity measurement of 0.33 centipoise (approximately one-third that of whole blood), transfusion of HBOC-201 also decreases the overall viscosity of a patient's blood, resulting in improvement in a patient in shock who already has constricted peripheral vasculature. In addition, by virtue of its P_{50} value of 43 mm Hg, HBOC-201 has a slight right shift, which promotes the delivery of oxygen to tissues compared with RBCs. These two key principles have been borne out in clinical studies that demonstrated an improvement in the efficiency of HBOC hemoglobin at delivering oxygen to tissues[8] and an ability to prevent or reduce tissue hypoxia.[9]

Various clinical studies have shown initial efficacy of HBOC-201. HBC-201 has been shown to eliminate the need for PRBC transfusion in 27% of patients undergoing elective aortic surgery[10] and in 34% of patients after coronary artery bypass.[11] To date, in healthy volunteers[12] and in a subgroup of patients undergoing hemodilution for elective abdominal surgery,[13] concerns about a sudden increase in systemic vascular resistance have dampened the initial enthusiasm that was seen after several animal studies of HBOC-201 showed promise in the treatment of hemorrhagic shock.[14]

Common to each of these products are recurrent concerns regarding adverse effects and fairly significant physiologic consequences that appear following administration. In one large animal study of 32 swine using a hemorrhagic shock model, resuscitation from a mean arterial pressure of 35 ± 5 mm Hg was undertaken with HBOC-201. Although mean arterial pressure and cardiac output returned to baseline with HBOC-201, unlike with lactated Ringer's and hypertonic saline, resuscitation was complicated by a significant increase in peripheral vascular resistance and mean pulmonary artery pressure.[15] Multiple other investigators have demonstrated this vasoconstriction and moderate to severe pulmonary hypertension, in addition to death, gastrointestinal symptoms, and other cardiac events.[16]

Although no single large study has definitively addressed these safety concerns, other investigators have continued to elucidate these risks specifically in trauma and surgical populations. Most recently, Natanson and colleagues[17] performed a meta-analysis of 16 trials involving five different HBOC products. Using a fixed-effects model, data from these trials were combined and evaluated. These combined results revealed a significant risk of myocardial infarction in the HBOC treatment group (relative risk [RR]: 2.71; 95% confidence interval [CI]: 1.67–4.40) and a significant increase in the risk of death (RR: 1.30; 95% CI: 1.05–1.61). Clearly, advanced clinical trials that are underway will need to show significant benefits/improvements in safety profiles before widespread Food and Drug Administration approval.[18]

CHARACTERISTICS OF STORED PACKED RED BLOOD CELLS

As with many improvements in the care of the critically ill and injured, the ability to store and transfuse RBCs has been driven by the need to care for wounded soldiers. From the first documented direct blood transfusion to the injured by the Frenchman Jean-Baptise Denis, improvements in technique and the development of the specialty of transfusion medicine have increased PRBC maximum storage time. Using an original storage medium of citrate anticoagulant and dextrose, the maximum storage time of PRBCs during World War I was approximately 14 days.[19] With the addition of cellular nutrients to the storage media, the maximum storage time has been increased to 42 days. Of interest, as described eloquently by Ho and colleagues[20] in their review article on the effects of storage on RBC efficacy and safety, apart from these changes made in the 1940s, the basic media and storage techniques remain the standard of practice today.

Storage of PRBCs outside of endothelial-lined spaces has always been a challenge. Only relatively recently have changes in the morphologic, physiologic, and biochemical properties of stored PRBCs been clearly elucidated to have less-than optimal effects on the patients into which they are transfused. Termed the "RBC storage defect,"[21] these problems have been implicated in a number of clinical problems in critically ill patients.

The RBC storage defect is defined primarily by alterations in the cellular morphology of the RBC itself, limiting its ability to traverse the microcirculation and deliver its oxygen content, and by changes in the storage medium.[9] The primary change in RBC morphology is a transition from a biconcave disc of approximately 8 μm in diameter, to more of a "spheroechinocyte" of considerably larger diameter.[22] Thought to be the result of diminished levels of ATP, these larger, misshapen PRBCs have difficulty traversing the 3- to 8-μm diameter microcirculation and can lead to decreased oxygen delivery to the periphery. In addition, decreases in 2,3-diphosphoglycerate levels in the stored RBC itself lead to increases in oxygen-affinity,[23] also decreasing oxygen delivery to the periphery in already anemic patients for whom the transfusion of PRBCs has been ordered.

In addition to the morphologic changes, detrimental changes in the storage medium of PRBCs are developed after long storage times. Breakdown of white blood cells over the storage period releases free radicals[24] and causes cell breakdown and potassium leakage.[25] Several of these changes, thought to be the result of white blood cell contamination of the PRBC product, have been mitigated by the prestorage leukoreduction that has become popular over the last several years.[26]

The previously described storage defect does not just exist in a test tube. It remains a real problem in the treatment of patients requiring PRBC transfusion. In trauma patients—one of the largest groups of consumers of PRBC transfusion in the United States—the transfusion of PRBCs older than 14 days has been implicated in increasing the incidence of postinjury multiple organ failure[27] and the risk of a postinjury major infectious complication.[28]

Other patient populations have also felt the effects of the RBC storage defect. In the postoperative cardiac surgery patient population, investigators have demonstrated an increased risk of pneumonia of 1% per day of mean PRBC storage time,[29] whereas other researchers have shown that increasing age of the oldest unit of transfused PRBC is an independent predictor of ventilator-associated pneumonia.[30] In patients who have severe sepsis, one study showed a significant decrease in survival to hospital discharge in those transfused with PRBCs greater than 16 days old,[31] whereas another study (a prospective, controlled trial) showed a clear decrease in gastric mucosal pH (a marker of splanchnic ischemia) after the transfusion of RBCs stored longer than 15 days.[32]

Although not specifically related to the storage defect, ABT has also been associated with a number of infectious and immune complications. A recent review on the topic described potential mechanisms of the blood transfusion–related immunomodulation associated with ABT.[33] These mechanisms included the transmission of immunologically active white blood cells that down-regulate the recipient's immune function, soluble immune modifiers accumulated during RBC storage, and soluble mediators that circulate in the small amount of plasma that is transfused with a unit of stored RBCs.

In addition, recent years have seen the definition and elucidation of these deleterious immune effects of ABT on specific organ systems. Transfusion-related acute lung injury (TRALI) has gone from an infrequently recognized, ill-defined rare event to the most common cause of transfusion-related morbidity. Originally defined clinically in 2004, TRALI includes the syndrome of posttransfusion respiratory distress, noncardiac pulmonary edema, and hypoxemia. Although the exact pathogenesis remains controversial, it is clear that neutrophil priming agents present in stored PRBC products are associated (at the least) and may be causative.[34]

HEMOGLOBIN-BASED OXYGEN CARRIERS VERSUS STORED RED BLOOD CELLS: IS THERE A RIGHT ANSWER?

In attempting a direct, head-to-head comparison, very little in the way of clinical literature exists to formulate a truly scientific opinion. Each therapy presently has strengths and weaknesses.

In terms of logistics, the HBOC group clearly has some potential advantages. The ability of Hemopure/HBOC-201 to be transported and stored for long periods of time without refrigeration and to be administered without any laboratory/blood bank testing to determine type/cross-match represents a significant advantage over stored PRBCs—an advantage that many military agencies are intending to attempt to exploit.[35] Presently, the United States military uses a specialized transport box for PRBCs and other blood components. Originally designed in 1965 and still in common use today, the Collins Box is a 3-cu ft, 40-lb box made of cardboard and capable of carrying 18 units of PRBCs cooled by wet ice.[36] Cumbersome and unwieldy, especially in areas of far-forward operations, PBRC transfusion and component therapy may be impossible in certain situations. In contrast, a few units of HBOC carried in the packs of far-forward deployed medics can be easily administered to wounded soldiers. Thus, the concept of HBOC as a "hemoglobin bridge" becomes very attractive.

Although HBOCs are undergoing continued development and are not yet readily available for clinical practice, many military surgeons have overcome the problem of transport/storage of blood component products and the RBC storage defect by using fresh, whole blood as a resuscitative fluid.[37] Termed the "walking blood bank," this practice has saved many lives during Operations Enduring Freedom and Iraqi Freedom. Volunteer donors, screened at the time of donation for hepatitis and HIV, donate a product that (1) encompasses many of today's blood component therapies, (2) is devoid of the storage medium and defect described earlier, and (3) is already warm at the time of administration without any additional warming.[38] Although not a viable option in other settings, the walking blood bank has served admirably during the country's most recent conflicts.

SUMMARY

Because of continued clinical concerns, it is clear that HBOCs as a substitute for the use of stored PRBCs are not yet ready for regular use in the clinical arena; however, as HBOC products continue to improve and become clinically available and as the elucidation of the mechanisms of their adverse effects becomes clearer, this may change in the near future. While this development continues, we must further the development of alternative strategies for the hemoglobin bridge so desperately needed by many critically ill patients.

REFERENCES

1. Spence RK, et al. Blood substitutes. In: Petz LD, Swisher SN, Kleinman S, editors. Clinical practice of transfusion medicine. 3rd edition. New York: Churchill Livingstone; 1996. p. 967–84.
2. Hess JR, Reiss RF. Resuscitation and the limited utility of present generation blood substitutes. Transfus Med Rev 1996;10:276–85.
3. Ketcham EM, Cairns CB. Hemoglobin-based oxygen carriers: development and clinical potential. Ann Emerg Med 1999;33(3):326–37.
4. Jahr JS, Walker V, Monoocheri K, et al. Blood substitutes as pharmacotherapies in clinical practice. Curr Opin Anaesthesiol 2007;20(4):325–30.
5. Hébert PC, Chin-Yee I, Fergusson D, et al. and the Canadian Critical Care Trials Group. A pilot trial evaluating the clinical effects of prolonged storage of red cells. Anesth Analg 2005;100:1433–58.
6. Nuttal GA, Brost BC, Connis RT, et al. Practice guidelines for perioperative blood transfusion and adjuvant therapies: an updated report by the American Society of Anesthesiologists Task Force on perioperative blood transfusion and adjuvant therapies. Anesthesiology 2006;105:198–208.
7. Gould SA, Moore EE, Hoyt DB, et al. The life-sustaining capacity of human polymerized hemoglobin when red cells might be unavailable. J Am Coll Surg 2002; 195:445–52.
8. Standl T, Horn P, Wilhelm S, et al. Bovine hemoglobin is more potent than autologus red blood cells in restoring muscular issue oxygenation after profound isovolaemic haemodilution in dogs. Can J Anaesth 1996;43(7):714–23.
9. Horn EP, Standl T, Wilhelm S, et al. Bovine hemoglobin increases skeletal muscle oxygenation during 95% artificial arterial stenosis. Surgery 1997;121(4):411–8.
10. LaMuraglia GM, O'Hara PJ, Baker WH, et al. The reduction of the allogeneic transfusion requirement in aortic surgery with a hemoglobin-based solution. J Vasc Surg 2000;31:299–308.
11. Levy JH, Goodnough LT, Greilich P, et al. Polymerized bovine hemoglobin solution as a replacement for allogeneic red blood cell transfusion: results of a randomized, double-blind trial. J Thorac Cardiovasc Surg 2002;124:35–42.

12. Hughes GS, Antal EJ, Locker PK, et al. Physiology and pharmacokinetics of a novel hemoglobin-based oxygen carrier in humans. Crit Care Med 1996;24: 756–64.
13. Kasper SM, Walter M, Grune F, et al. Effects of a hemoglobin-based oxygen carrier (HBOC-201) on hemodynamics and oxygen transport in patients undergoing preoperative hemodilution for elective abdominal aortic surgery. Anesth Analg 1996;83:921–7.
14. McNeil JD, Smith DL, Jenkins DH, et al. Hypotensive resuscitation using a polymerized bovine-based oxygen carrying solution leads to reversal of anaerobic metabolism. J Trauma 2001;50:1063–75.
15. Rivera-Chavez FA, Huerta S, et al. Resuscitation from hemorrhagic shock comparing standard hemoglobin-based oxygen carrier (HBOC)-201 versus 7.5% hypertonic HBOC-201. J Trauma 2007;63(5):1113–9.
16. Winslow RM. Red cell substitutes. Semin Hematol 2007;44:51–9.
17. Natanson C, Kern SJ, Lurie P, et al. Cell-free hemoglobin-based blood substitutes and risk of myocardial infarction and death. JAMA 2008;299(19): 2304–12.
18. Winslow RM. Blood substitutes: basic principles and practical aspects. In: Hillyer CD, editor. Blood banking and transfusion medicine. Basic principles and practice. St. Louis (MO): Churchill Livingstone; 2007.
19. Landsteiner K, Levine P. Note on individual differences in human blood. Proc Soc Exp Biol Med 1931;28:309.
20. Ho J, Sibbald WJ, Chin-Yee IH. Effects of storage on efficacy of red-cell transfusion: when is it not safe? Crit Care Med 2003;31(12):s687–97.
21. Tinmouth A, Chin-Yee I. The clinical consequences of the red cell storage lesion. Transfus Med Rev 2001;15:91–107.
22. Nakao M, Nakao T, Yamazoes S, et al. Adenosine triphosphate and maintenance of shape of human red cells. Nature 1960;187:945–6.
23. Valtis DJ, Kennedy AC. Defective gas-transport function of stored red blood cells. Lancet 1954;1:119–25.
24. Chin-Yee I, d'Almeida MS. A comparison of biochemical and functional alterations of rat and human erythrocytes stored in CDPA-1 for 29 days: implications for animal models of transfusion. Transfus Med 2000;10:291–303.
25. Hogman CFR, Meryman HT. Storage parameters affecting red blood cell survival and function after transfusion. Transfus Med Rev 1999;13:275–96.
26. Plurad D, Belzberg H, Schulman I, et al. Leukoreduction is associated with a decreased incidence of late onset acute respiratory distress syndrome after injury. Am Surg 2008;74(2):117–23.
27. Zallen G, Offner PJ, Moore EE, et al. Age of transfused blood is an independent risk factor for postinjury multiple organ failure. Am J Surg 1999;178: 570–2.
28. Offner PJ, Moore EE, Biffl WL, et al. Increased rate of infection associated with transfusion of old blood after severe injury. Arch Surg 2002;137:711–7.
29. Vamvakas EC, Carven JH. Transfusion and postoperative pneumonia in coronary artery bypass graft surgery: effect of the length of storage of transfused red cells. Transfusion 1999;39:701–10.
30. Leal-Noval SR, Jara-Lopez I, Garcia-Garmendia JL, et al. Influence of erythrocyte concentrate storage time on postsurgical morbidity in cardiac surgery patients. Anesthesiology 2003;98:815–22.
31. Purdy FR, Tweeddale MG, Merrick PM, et al. Association of mortality with age of blood transfused in septic ICU patients. Can J Anaesth 1997;44:1256–61.

32. Marik PE, Sibbald WJ. Effect of stored-blood transfusion on oxygen delivery in patients with sepsis. JAMA 1993;269:3024–9.
33. Gunst MA, Minei JP. Transfusion of blood products and nosocomial infection in surgical patients. Curr Opin Crit Care 2007;13:428–32.
34. Bux J, Sachs UJ. The pathogenesis of transfusion-related acute lung injury (TRALI). Br J Haematol 2007;136(6):788–99.
35. Ness PM, Cushing MD. Oxygen therapeutics. Pursuit of an alternative to the donor red blood cell. Arch Pathol Lab Med 2007;131:734–41.
36. Rentas FJ, Macdonald VW, Houchens DM, et al. New insulation technology provides next-generation containers for 'iceless' and lightweight transport of RBCs at 1 to 10°C in extreme temperatures for over 78 h. Transfusion 2004;44: 210–6.
37. Kauvar DS, Holcomb JB, Norris GC, et al. Fresh whole blood transfusion: a controversial military practice. J Trauma 2006;61:181–4.
38. Sebesta J. Special lessons learned from Iraq. Surg Clin North Am 2006;86: 711–26.

Potential Uses of Hemoglobin-based Oxygen Carriers in Critical Care Medicine

Jacques Creteur, MD, PhD, Jean-Louis Vincent, MD, PhD*

KEYWORDS

- Oncotic pressure • Nitric oxide • Sepsis
- Perioperative blood loss • Transfusion
- Oxygen transport • Red blood cell • Trauma

The two major impulses driving the development of hemoglobin-based oxygen carriers (HBOCs) are concerns about the infectious risks of transfusion and worries about limitations in the availability of blood. Almost 40,000 red blood cell (RBC) transfusions are given each day in the United States, and about 5 million Americans receive transfusions every year for a variety of reasons. The volume of blood transfused is increasing at the rate of 6% per year, and the greatest fear of the blood bank community at present is impending shortages. Although seasonal and regional shortages are not uncommon, an extended, nationwide shortage of blood has not been observed in recent history, even though about 6% of United States hospitals have reported that surgical procedures have had to be cancelled or postponed because of blood shortages.[1] A shortage of RBCs may occur, however, if transfusion demand continues to increase and if collections cannot keep pace.[1]

Considerable progress has been made in developing HBOC products that meet many of the criteria for a clinically useful and safe oxygen carrier, including better shelf stability than banked RBCs, universal compatibility, useful vascular half-life, and absence of infectious agents (**Box 1**). The HBOCs under development all have vascular half-lives in the 18- to 24-hour range, which is adequate for most acute-care applications (ie, hemorrhage and surgery); most can be stored at 4°C or room temperature for 1 to 2 years; and none requires any form of compatibility testing. All the HBOCs currently developed have been successfully processed to eliminate the presence of microorganisms, although there are very few published data on the removal of prions.

With the realization that HBOCs not only are RBC substitutes but also have many other properties, including hemodynamic effects related to their oncotic and nitric

Department of Intensive Care, Erasme Hospital, Université libre de Bruxelles, Route de Lennik 808, 1070 Brussels, Belgium
* Corresponding author.
E-mail address: jlvincen@ulb.ac.be (J-L. Vincent).

Crit Care Clin 25 (2009) 311–324
doi:10.1016/j.ccc.2008.12.011
0749-0704/08/$ – see front matter © 2009 Elsevier Inc. All rights reserved.

criticalcare.theclinics.com

Box 1
Potential advantages of HBOCs over RBC transfusion

No antigenicity—universally compatible

Possible unlimited availability (animal or recombinant source)

No disease-transmission risk

Long storage life

---

oxide (NO)-scavenging effects, a new, broader concept of "hemoglobin therapeutics" has developed. HBOCs, therefore, are now seen as a complement to RBC transfusions, not a replacement. The present review focuses on the potential uses of HBOCs in critical care medicine.

PROPERTIES OF HEMOGLOBIN-BASED OXYGEN CARRIERS
Oxygen-Carrying Capacity

Hemoglobin concentration, hemoglobin saturation, and blood flow are key determinants of tissue oxygen availability, so strategies to increase systemic oxygen transport (convective oxygen transport—ie, circulation) are usually employed when attempting to increase tissue oxygen availability. Nevertheless, these factors are not the only determinants of tissue oxygenation in critical illness.[2] Sepsis is characterized by microcirculatory alterations[3] that can lead to tissue hypoxia, despite the presence of elevated convective oxygen transport. Even with a high oxygen-carrying capacity, a solution that alters the microcirculation is not efficient at improving tissue oxygenation. The different types of HBOCs have very different hemodynamic properties (vasoconstrictive and oncotic effects), so their effects on the microcirculation may be very different. In theory, a small amount of a hemoglobin solution with no vasopressor effects is more effective in improving tissue oxygenation than a large amount of a vasopressor solution that alters microcirculatory blood flow. Nevertheless, in general, compared with nonhemoglobin solutions, resuscitation fluids containing hemoglobin improve oxygen transport to the tissues.[4–10]

Oncotic Effects

RBCs have a negligible effect on the colloid osmotic pressure (COP). HBOCs, however, exert substantial oncotic properties and thus increase blood volume by an amount greater than the transfused volume.[11] This action may be beneficial when plasma expansion is required in shock resuscitation but can also be harmful in the absence of hypovolemia. It has been proposed that hyperoncotic HBOCs may decrease ischemic brain injury.[12] Nevertheless, the beneficial effects of a reduction in blood viscosity on microvascular blood flow may also be important. Using bioengineering analysis and novel methods to measure intravascular and tissue Po_2, Intaglietta and colleagues[13] proposed that maintaining the viscosity of blood (~ 4 centipoise) is essential to maintain tissue oxygenation. Indeed, the relation between blood viscosity and vascular relaxation is explained by the fact that the shear forces exerted on endothelial cells are proportional to blood viscosity, and these shear forces induce the production of the vasodilator, NO.[14,15] Tsai and colleagues[16] showed that deep hemodilution with high viscosity dextran maintained functional capillary density in the hamster skin-fold model significantly better than with low viscosity dextran. These discoveries force a re-evaluation of the optimal viscosity of an RBC substitute. It was formerly thought that such a solution should have a low viscosity to reduce peripheral vascular resistance and to elevate cardiac output; now, the opposite appears to be the case.

Vasopressor Effects

Many experimental studies have reported a rise in blood pressure following the administration of HBOCs,[5,7,10,17–22] and clinical trials have confirmed this observation.[9,23–29] These vasopressor effects are, at least in part, due to the scavenging of NO.[19,30–35] The NO-scavenging effects may be mitigated by encapsulating the hemoglobin in liposomes, because these larger molecules have less contact with the endothelium and are less able to penetrate the endothelium to combine with NO.[36] Endothelin-1, a strong vasoconstrictor produced by endothelial cells and acting directly on vascular smooth muscle, may also be involved in the vasoconstrictor effects of hemoglobin solutions.[22,31,37,38] Nevertheless, effects other than NO scavenging must be involved. Indeed, some investigators[39] have demonstrated that various types of modified hemoglobins (cross-linked, polymerized, or surface-modified) elicit various blood pressure responses that are inversely related to the size of the hemoglobin molecule but not to the degree of reactivity with NO. Sakai and colleagues[40] studied the effects of different HBOCs of various molecular sizes on the diameter of resistance arteries and arterial blood pressure in the conscious hamster dorsal skin-fold model. These investigators found that the vasoconstrictive response of resistance arteries was correlated with the degree of hypertension and that the responses were proportional to the molecular dimensions of the oxygen carriers. These observations are best explained by the relation between molecular size, oxyhemoglobin diffusion, and vasoconstriction. It has long been known that oxyhemoglobin can diffuse along a concentration gradient, a process called "facilitated diffusion."[41,42] It has been proposed that this oxygen availability could be significantly increased by free plasma hemoglobin. One group of investigators showed that administration of such an HBOC increased pulmonary diffusing capacity.[9] At first glance, this facilitated oxygen transfer might be considered beneficial; however, direct observation of the microcirculation has shown that precapillary arterioles are very sensitive to local oxygen concentration, enabling them to adjust their diameter in an autoregulatory process to increase capillary blood flow in hypoxia and to decrease it in hyperoxia.[43] Using direct measurement of the diffusive oxygen transfer by hemoglobin in an artificial capillary system, McCarthy and colleagues[44] confirmed the link between molecular size, diffusion, and vasoconstriction. These investigators demonstrated that the rate of oxygen transfer out of the in vitro microvessel was higher with cross-linked hemoglobin than with larger-size surface-modified hemoglobin, such as polyethylene glycol (PEG)-modified bovine hemoglobin (PEG-Hb), which has negligible vasoactive effects.[39,45] Indeed, Winslow and colleagues[45] compared the effects of PEG-Hb (high oxygen affinity, high viscosity, high COP) with human hemoglobin cross-linked between the α-chains ($\alpha\alpha$-Hb; low oxygen affinity, low viscosity, low COP) after a 50% (by volume) exchange transfusion followed by severe hemorrhage in rats. The investigators found that mean arterial pressure and systemic vascular resistance rose significantly in the $\alpha\alpha$-Hb but not in the PEG-Hb animals. In addition, the PEG-Hb animals showed no acid-base disturbance, significantly less lactic acidosis, and a higher cardiac output. These data suggest that the rise in vascular resistance that follows the $\alpha\alpha$-Hb exchange transfusion offsets the greater oxygen transport provided by the cell-free hemoglobin. When resistance does not rise, as with PEG-Hb, even relatively small amounts of cell-free hemoglobin appear to provide very effective blood replacement. Such beneficial effects of a hemoglobin solution on the microcirculation were demonstrated by Wettstein and colleagues,[46] who resuscitated hamsters from severe hemorrhagic shock with a new PEG-modified human hemoglobin solution—malPEG-Hb, an oxygen-carrying blood replacement fluid with low hemoglobin concentration, high viscosity, high COP, and very low P50 (5 mm Hg). Compared with resuscitation with shed blood or colloid, the infusion of malPEG-Hb was followed by an improvement in microcirculatory blood flow (increased functional capillary density) and microcirculatory oxygen extraction capabilities, resulting in a complete reversal of metabolic acidosis. This result was not seen in animals resuscitated with shed blood or colloid, even though the total plasma hemoglobin concentration was lower in the malPEG-Hb than in the shed blood group. Again, this study[46] seems to underline the efficacy of a solution that associates high viscosity, high COP, and high oxygen affinity properties to maintain microvascular blood flow and tissue oxygenation. In this case, even a low-dose oxygen carrier may be superior to autologous blood in returning the organism to normal conditions after hemorrhagic shock.[46] Properties of first- and second-generation HBOCs are summarized in **Table 1**.

USE OF HEMOGLOBIN-BASED OXYGEN CARRIERS AS A BLOOD SUBSTITUTE

A blood substitute that eliminates the need for refrigeration and cross-matching, that has a long shelf life, and that reduces the risk of iatrogenic infection would provide a potentially lifesaving option for trauma patients who have hemorrhagic shock, especially in rural areas and military settings. For their use in the hospital, blood substitute HBOCs should be at least as safe as RBCs transfusions, even though the risks associated with transfusion have become relatively low in developed countries. At locations where RBCs are not immediately available, the risks of HBOCs need to be balanced against those of resuscitation fluids. One topic of active debate over the past decade was the definition of "efficacy" of HBOCs. Demonstrating survival benefit in most clinical models is very challenging, and correlating oxygen delivery and other variables with survival outcome is equally difficult. Therefore, avoidance of allogeneic transfusion has almost become a universal marker of efficacy for these solutions in clinical trials.

Trauma and Hemorrhagic Shock

Because of their hemodynamic properties (see earlier discussion), HBOCs would appear to be ideal solutions for initial resuscitation from trauma or hemorrhage in the emergency room and even in the field. Gould and colleagues[47] compared the therapeutic benefit of PolyHeme (a human polymerized hemoglobin; Northfield Laboratories, Inc., Evanston, Illinois) with that of allogeneic RBCs in the treatment of acute blood loss in trauma patients. PolyHeme maintained total hemoglobin concentration despite the fall in RBC hemoglobin, and reduced the use of allogeneic blood. Later, PolyHeme was studied by the same group in massively bleeding trauma and urgent surgery patients who did not receive RBCs.[48] A total of 171 patients received a rapid

Table 1		
Properties of first- and second-generation hemoglobin-based oxygen carriers		
Property	**First Generation**	**Second-Generation**
Oxygen binding	Like blood: P50 $\pm$28 mm Hg	P50 $\pm$5–10 mm Hg
Viscosity	Like water: $\pm$1 centipoise	Like blood: $\pm$4 centipoise
Oncotic pressure	Like blood: $\pm$15 mm Hg	Increased
Hemoglobin concentration	Like blood: $\pm$15 g/dL	As low as possible
Plasma retention	As long as possible	As long as possible
Clinical use	Substitute for RBCs	Hemoglobin therapeutics

infusion of 1 to 20 units (1000 g, 10 L) of PolyHeme. Forty patients had a nadir RBC hemoglobin below 3 g/dL, but total hemoglobin was adequately maintained (6.8 ± 0.7 g/dL) by the plasma hemoglobin added by PolyHeme. The 30-day mortality was 25% compared with 64% in a historical group of control patients who had similar RBC hemoglobin levels. Less encouraging were the results of the pivotal phase III trauma trial with the Baxter Healthcare Corporation (Baxter) diaspirin cross-linked hemoglobin (DCLHb) product.[49] This United States multicenter trial was designed to determine whether the infusion of up to 1000 mL of DCLHb during initial hospital resuscitation could reduce 28-day mortality in traumatic hemorrhage. The study was stopped prematurely after the enrolment of 112 patients when an intermediate analysis showed an increased 28-day mortality in the DCLHb-resuscitated group compared with the control group (46 versus 17%, respectively; $P = .003$). The investigators could not correlate the excessive mortality with any specific morbidity but reported that the DCLHb treatment group showed a higher incidence of prehospital cardiac arrest and traumatic brain injuries. They concluded that the vasopressor effect could have contributed to the untoward effect of DCLHb treatment, either by accelerating bleeding or by tissue vasoconstriction, both of which would decrease tissue perfusion. Baxter conducted a companion phase III trauma trial in Europe using morbidity, rather than mortality, as the efficacy end point.[50] Another important difference was that in the European study, the patients were already randomized "on the scene" to receive DCLHb or standard fluid therapy. Organ failures and survival rates until day 5 and day 28 showed no significant differences. The median volumes of cumulative blood products administered on day 1 (1595 versus 3716 mL) and day 7 (3139 versus 4746 mL) were lower in the DCLHb group than in the control group. The trial, however, was discontinued after 121 of the expected 400 to 800 patients were enrolled because Baxter terminated the program. Nevertheless, it should be noted that the properties of DCLHb (and particularly the strong vasopressor effect) are not applicable to all HBOCs. Northfield Laboratories last year reported results of its pivotal phase III trauma trial with PolyHeme[51] on 30-day mortality in traumatic shock. Severely injured patients were randomized at the scene to receive PolyHeme or crystalloid. The study group received up to 6 units (in the field or during the first 12 hours of hospitalization) of PolyHeme, followed by RBC transfusions as needed. The study was designed to have sufficient statistical power to demonstrate superiority and noninferiority end points. The secondary end points included incidence of multiple organ failure and avoidance of blood transfusion. The study population consisted of 722 patients at more than 30 trauma centers throughout the United States. Only preliminary results from the trial have been reported by Northfield Laboratories in the press:[51] mortality at 30 days was not statistically different in control patients compared with those treated with PolyHeme (9.6 versus 13.4%). The results of these studies should be considered in the context of bleeding patients for whom early access to blood transfusion is not possible. Even in the United States, almost 50 million Americans live more than an hour away from a trauma center where blood is available. Mortality rates in such a scenario could be considerably higher than those observed in the control patients in the urban setting of the studies discussed earlier, for whom transit times were relatively short. If these data are extrapolated to patients who need an oxygen carrier and have delayed access to blood, HBOCs such as PolyHeme could play an important role in saving lives.

Perioperative Blood Losses

Given the concerns about transfusion-related illness and the general fear of transfusions by the public and physicians, it is common for patients to ask for alternatives to banked blood. Almost all of the paradigms and algorithms for avoiding transfusion tend to be resource intense and expensive, and still do not eliminate all risk. Alternatives can be sought, and the use of HBOCs as part of intraoperative autologous donation makes a great deal of sense. HBOCs may also be valuable during the perioperative period when blood is often transfused in small quantities to maximize the patient's oxygen-carrying capacity and to replace normal expected surgical blood loss. It is clear that blood substitutes will never be able to completely replace entire circulating blood volume. They might, therefore, be considered more a "bridge" until blood transfusion is available or be used to avoid RBC transfusion altogether when blood losses are moderate. Cross-linked[26,52] and polymerized hemoglobin[27-29,53,54] have shown efficacy in several studies (in cardiac[26-28,53,54] and noncardiac[29,52] surgery) that used blood sparing in the perioperative period as the efficacy end point. These studies showed a subsequent reduction in RBC transfusions at 24 hours; however, due to the short half-life of these products, this effect was transient. The adverse effects encountered in these different studies were transient increases in blood pressure, jaundice, and transient, mild increases in enzyme levels that were not obviously related to pathologic liver dysfunction or pancreatitis. Nevertheless, one of these studies was terminated early because of these safety concerns.[52] In two small studies of patients before[55] and after[56] repair of abdominal aortic aneurysm, DCLHb was associated with a decrease in cardiac output due to an increase in afterload, which may pose a serious problem in patients who have altered left ventricular function. Of note, one patient treated with DCLHb had a myocardial infarction 36 hours post infusion.[56] Olofsson and colleagues[57] conducted a safety phase II study in patients undergoing major orthopedic study. These investigators compared Ringer's acetate with two different doses of Hemospan (Sangart, Inc., San Diego, California) given before the induction of anesthesia. Hemospan mildly elevated hepatic enzymes and lipase and was associated with less hypotension and more bradycardic events. A randomized controlled, multicenter phase III trial using a polymerized bovine hemoglobin (Hemopure; Biopure Corporation, Cambridge, Massachusetts) in elective orthopedic surgery was completed in the United States in which 350 patients received Hemopure and 338 received RBC transfusions. The investigators reported that 59.4% of the patients receiving Hemopure were able to avoid allogeneic RBC transfusions; mortality and serious adverse events were comparable in the two treatment groups.[58]

Polymerized bovine hemoglobin (Hemopure) received regulatory approval in South Africa in 2001 for clinical use in the treatment of acute anemia and the avoidance of allogeneic blood transfusion during surgery in adults. Nevertheless, a recent meta-analysis[59] showed that the administration of HBOCs in patients who had surgery, trauma, or stroke was associated with a significant risk of myocardial infarction and death. The meta-analysis of 16 clinical trials with five very different HBOCs showed that administration of any of the products was associated with a higher relative risk of death and of heart attack than was observed in the control groups in the trials; however, the limitation of this analysis was the pooling of very different products used in different settings against different comparators. Some of these products have been withdrawn from development and some of the respective companies have since gone out of business.

Another potential benefit of HBOCs would be in the patient who has multiple antibodies to RBC surface antigens because of multiple previous transfusions and who risks serious transfusion reactions if further RBC transfusion were required. Finally, the recombinant technology could theoretically offer a new therapeutic option in the management of Jehovah's Witness patients.

USE OF HEMOGLOBIN-BASED OXYGEN CARRIERS AS "HEMOGLOBIN THERAPEUTICS"
Sepsis and Septic Shock

Sepsis is characterized by profound microcirculatory alterations.[3,60] With their potentially favorable rheologic properties, HBOCs may increase tissue oxygen availability and oxygen extraction capacity. In septic rats, Sielenkämper and colleagues[61] demonstrated a beneficial effect of DCLHb on tissue oxygen use. When oxygen supply dependency was induced by progressive hemodilution, DCLHb infusion increased oxygen uptake and reversed lactic acidosis. The authors also studied the effects of DCLHb on blood flow distribution and tissue oxygen extraction capabilities in a canine model of endotoxic shock.[62] DCLHb had a dose-dependent vasopressor effect but did not significantly alter cardiac index or regional blood flow. The administration of DCLHb was also followed by an improvement in whole-body oxygen-extraction capabilities.

During sepsis, an increase in inducible NO synthase (NOS) activation leads to overproduction of NO, which is thought to play a role in the pathogenesis of associated hypotension.[63–65] Blockers of NOS activity in animal and clinical studies attenuate these pressure-related effects;[66] however, excessive NO blockade can be harmful,[67] and the use of HBOCs may provide an alternative means of restoring blood pressure and oxygen-extraction capabilities by scavenging NO rather than by entirely blocking NO production. Infusion of pyridoxylated hemoglobin polyoxyethylene (PHP) conjugate in endotoxemic sheep has been shown to have less effect on cardiac index and pulmonary vascular resistance than NOS inhibition with NG-nitro-L-arginine methyl ester.[68] In other studies, HBOC solutions showed protective effects on the kidney by the combined effects of volume expansion and inactivation of NO.[17,69,70] In experimental sepsis, HBOCs have also been shown to prevent myocardial dysfunction.[71,72] In summary, compared with harmful total NO blockade, the use of HBOCs to scavenge NO may provide an alternative means of restoring blood pressure and oxygen-extraction capabilities without entirely blocking NO activity. In a small preliminary study of 14 patients in septic shock, DCLHb infusion allowed a reduction in vasopressor needs to support systemic blood pressure.[25] Nevertheless, this vasopressor effect was accompanied by a reduction in cardiac index and oxygen delivery.[25] A transient increase in total plasma bilirubin was also observed in patients treated with DCLHb.[25]

Recently, Apex Bioscience (Chapel Hill, North Carolina) announced the termination of a study assessing the safety and efficacy of PHP in patients who have distributive shock. This study was a placebo-controlled, randomized, open label study at 15 sites that was initially designed to enroll 1000 patients. The study was terminated early, at 62 patients, because of a protocol design issue (about 800 screen failures due to the absence of a pulmonary artery catheter in situ, an inclusion criterion for the study). Recently published results[73] noted that overall 28-day mortality was similar in the group of patients treated with PHP and in the control group. Nevertheless, survivors treated with PHP tended to be weaned off vasopressors faster and to spend less time on mechanical ventilation.

Although HBOCs may provide an alternative means of restoring blood pressure, improving cellular oxygen availability, and scavenging excess NO release, the potentially deleterious immunomodulatory effects of such solutions in sepsis must be considered. The preparation of these solutions is safe with respect to viral transmission, but because hemoglobin provides an important source of iron, which is necessary to sustain rapid multiplication and growth of bacteria, concerns have been raised about the possibility that hemoglobin solutions could promote infection.[74] Free hemoglobin can also abolish the bactericidal and bacteriostatic effects of plasma and inactivate neutrophils.[75] Griffiths and colleagues[76] reported that after sublethal *Escherichia coli* challenge in an experimental peritonitis model in mice, survival was reduced after a large intravenous dose of modified hemoglobin solution. Su and colleagues[77] reported that αα-Hb intensified the tumor necrosis factor response to lipopolysaccharide and that mortality after lipopolysaccharide injection was increased in αα-Hb–pretreated mice compared with control mice. The metabolism of these modified hemoglobins may also pose a problem, because their entrapment by macrophages may result in rapid saturation of the reticuloendothelial system, leading to a potential immunodepressant effect. Finally, free iron derived from hemoglobin breakdown can catalyze the production of oxygen free radicals, and the uptake of hemoglobin or ferruginous debris by macrophages may amplify the proinflammatory response, thereby increasing the release of cytokines such as tumor necrosis factor.[78–80] Liposome encapsulation may prevent this phenomenon.[81,82] Promising effects of HBOCs on oxygen transport and the microcirculation in sepsis need to be confirmed, and results from continuing research are eagerly awaited.

Stroke and Myocardial Infarction

Despite promising results in experimental models,[83–85] DCLHb has not been shown to be safe in patients who have cerebral infarction. Saxena and colleagues[86] assessed the safety and tolerability of DCLHb started within 18 hours of symptom onset in patients who had acute ischemic stroke. DCLHb caused a rapid rise in mean arterial pressure. Two patients infused with the high dose of DCLHb (100 mg/kg) had adverse events that were possibly drug related: one suffered fatal brain and pulmonary edema, the other experienced transient renal and pancreatic insufficiency. Multivariate logistic regression analysis showed that DCLHb treatment was an independent predictor of a worse outcome (odds ratio 4.0; confidence interval: 1.4–12.0).

Several experimental studies have demonstrated that HBOCs could preserve myocardial function and reduce infarct size after acute myocardial ischemia[87] by reducing ischemia-reperfusion injury.[88,89]

Sickle Cell Anemia

Patients who have sickle cell anemia comprise a unique population that might receive added benefits from HBOCs. These patients tend to be chronically transfused and also seem to be at a higher risk for becoming alloimmunized per unit transfused compared with the general population. The universal compatibility of HBOCs would be ideal to protect these patients from further alloimmunization and the risks of delayed hemolytic transfusion reactions. In addition, the availability of blood for sickle cell patients requiring phenotyped RBCs would be improved. HBOCs could be useful as urgent therapy for acute chest syndrome or other emergency vaso-occlusive events. These solutions may be useful to bridge patients who are alloimmunized until compatible blood can be found. There are a number of case reports in the literature of sickle cell patients who have benefited from HBOCs.[90–92] Although results from case reports are dramatic, larger studies with appropriate controls are required to verify these intriguing findings.

SUMMARY

Hemoglobin solutions were initially developed with the hope of finding an alternative to the problems associated with blood transfusion; however, with the realization that hemoglobin solutions not only are RBC substitutes but also have a number of additional properties, a new, broader concept of hemoglobin therapeutics developed.

Promising effects on oxygen transport and the microcirculation need to be confirmed, and the results of continuing research are eagerly awaited. Although debatable, the results of a recent meta-analysis[59] showing that the administration of HBOCs in surgical, stroke, and trauma patients was associated with a significant risk of myocardial infarction and death remind us that no drug is perfect or without side effects, and HBOCs are no exception. Today, we know the effects of the first generation of HBOCs. One area of interest is the development of new molecular structures to decrease NO binding so as to minimize the adverse consequences and to maximize the potential benefits. It is also fascinating to speculate that the choice among the various available solutions, with their different oxygen affinities, oxygen-carrying capacities, viscosities, and oncotic pressures, may be guided by clinical circumstances. Nevertheless, possible adverse effects need to be carefully evaluated before these agents can be widely administered in the ICU, emergency room, or prehospital setting.

REFERENCES

1. Winslow RM. Blood substitutes: refocusing an elusive goal. Br J Haematol 2000; 111:387–96.
2. Wagner PD. An integrated view of the determinants of maximum oxygen uptake. In: Gonzales NC, Fredde MR, editors. Oxygen transfer from atmosphere to tissues. New York: Plenum; 1988. p. 245–56.
3. De Backer D, Creteur J, Preiser JC, et al. Microvascular blood flow is altered in patients with sepsis. Am J Respir Crit Care Med 2002;166:98–104.
4. Vlahakes GJ, Lee R, Jacobs EE, et al. Hemodynamic effects and oxygen transport properties of a new blood substitute in a model of massive blood replacement. J Thorac Cardiovasc Surg 1990;100:379–88.
5. Przybelski RJ, Malcolm DS, Burris DG, et al. Cross-linked hemoglobin solution as a resuscitative fluid after hemorrhage in the rat. J Lab Clin Med 1991;117: 143–51.
6. Cohn SM, Farrell TJ. Diaspirin cross-linked hemoglobin resuscitation of hemorrhage: comparison of a blood substitute with hypertonic saline and isotonic saline. J Trauma 1994;39:210–7.
7. Lee R, Neya K, Svizzero TA, et al. Limitations of the efficacy of hemoglobin-based oxygen-carrying solutions. J Appl Physiol 1995;79:236–42.
8. Leppäniemi A, Soltero R, Burris D, et al. Early resuscitation with low-volume poly-DCLHb is effective in the treatment of shock induced by penetrating vascular injury. J Trauma 1996;40:242–8.
9. Hughes GS Jr, Antal EJ, Locker PK, et al. Physiology and pharmacokinetics of a novel hemoglobin-based oxygen carrier in humans. Crit Care Med 1996;24: 756–64.
10. Kerger H, Tsai AG, Saltzman DJ, et al. Fluid resuscitation with O_2 vs. non-O_2 carriers after 2h of hemorrhagic shock in conscious hamsters. Am J Physiol 1997;272:H525–37.
11. Migita R, Gonzales A, Gonzales ML, et al. Blood volume and cardiac index in rats after exchange transfusion with hemoglobin-based oxygen carriers. J Appl Physiol 1997;82:1995–2002.
12. Cole DJ, Drummond JC, Patel PM, et al. Effect of oncotic pressure of diaspirin cross-linked hemoglobin (DCLHb) on brain injury after temporary focal cerebral ischemia in rats. Anesth Analg 1996;83:342–7.

13. Intaglietta M, Johnson PC, Winslow RM. Microvascular and tissue oxygen distribution. Cardiovasc Res 1996;32:632–43.
14. Kuchan MJ, Frangos JA. Shear stress regulates endothelin-1 release via protein kinase C and cGMP in cultured endothelial cells. Am J Physiol 1993;264: H150–6.
15. Kuchan MJ, Jo H, Frangos JA. Role of G proteins in shear stress-mediated nitric oxide production by endothelial cells. Am J Physiol 1994;267:C753–8.
16. Tsai AG, Friesenecker B, McCarthy M, et al. Plasma viscosity regulates capillary perfusion during extreme hemodilution in hamster skinfold model. Am J Physiol 1998;275:H2170–80.
17. Thompson A, McGarry AE, Valeri CR, et al. Stroma-free hemoglobin increases blood pressure and GFR in the hypotensive rat: role of nitric oxide. J Appl Physiol 1994;77:2348–54.
18. Sharma AC, Gulati A. Effect of diaspirin cross-linked hemoglobin and norepinephrine on systemic hemodynamics and regional circulation in rats. J Lab Clin Med 1994;123:299–308.
19. Sharma AC, Singh G, Gulati A. Role of NO mechanism in cardiovascular effects of diaspirin cross-linked hemoglobin in anesthetized rats. Am J Physiol 1995;269: H1379–88.
20. Hindman BJ, Dexter F, Cutkomp J, et al. Diaspirin cross-linked hemoglobin dos not increase brain oxygen consumption during hypothermic cardiopulmonary bypass in rabbits. Anesthesiology 1995;83:1302–11.
21. Aranow JS, Wang H, Zhuang J, et al. Effect of human hemoglobin on systemic and regional hemodynamics in a porcine model of endotoxemic shock. Crit Care Med 1996;24:807–14.
22. Gulati A, Sharma AC, Singh G. Role of endothelin in the cardiovascular effects of diaspirin crosslinked and stroma reduced hemoglobin. Crit Care Med 1996;24: 137–47.
23. Kasper SM, Grune F, Walter M, et al. The effects of increased doses of bovine hemoglobin on hemodynamics and oxygen transport in patients undergoing preoperative hemodilution for elective abdominal aortic surgery. Anesth Analg 1998;87:284–91.
24. Przybelski RJ, Daily EK, Kisicki JC, et al. Phase I study of the safety and pharmacologic effects of diaspirin cross-linked hemoglobin solution. Crit Care Med 1996; 24:1993–2000.
25. Reah G, Bodenham AR, Mallick A, et al. Initial evaluation of diaspirin cross-linked hemoglobin (DCLHb) as a vasopressor in critically ill patients. Crit Care Med 1997;25:1480–8.
26. Lamy ML, Daily EK, Brichant JF, et al. Randomized trial of diaspirin cross-linked hemoglobin solution as an alternative to blood transfusion after cardiac surgery. Anesthesiology 2000;92:646–56.
27. Hill SE, Gottschalk LI, Grichnik K. Safety and preliminary efficacy of hemoglobin raffimer for patients undergoing coronary artery bypass surgery. J Cardiothorac Vasc Anesth 2002;16:695–702.
28. Levy JH, Goodnough LT, Greilich PE, et al. Polymerized bovine hemoglobin solution as a replacement for allogeneic red blood cell transfusion after cardiac surgery: results of a randomized, double-blind trial. J Thorac Cardiovasc Surg 2002;124:35–42.
29. LaMuraglia GM, O'Hara PJ, Baker WH, et al. The reduction of the allogenic transfusion requirement in aortic surgery with a hemoglobin-based solution. J Vasc Surg 2000;31:299–308.

30. Rooney MW, Hirsch LJ, Mathru M. Hemodilution with oxyhemoglobin: mechanism of oxygen deivery and its superaugmentation with a nitric oxide donor (sodium nitroprusside). Anesthesiology 1993;79:60–72.
31. Schultz SC, Grady B, Cole F, et al. A role for endothelin and nitric oxide in the pressor response to diaspirin cross-linked hemoglobin. J Lab Clin Med 1993; 122:301–8.
32. Freas W, Llave R, Jing M, et al. Contractile effects of diaspirin cross-linked hemoglobin (DCLHb) on isolated porcine blood vessels. J Lab Clin Med 1995;125: 762–7.
33. Ulatowski JA, Nishikawa T, Matheson-Urbaitis B, et al. Regional blood flow alterations after bovine fumaryl ββ-crosslinked hemoglobin transfusion and nitric oxide synthase inhibition. Crit Care Med 1996;24:558–65.
34. Hart JL, Ledvina MA, Muldoon SM. Actions of diaspirin cross-linked hemoglobin on isolated rat and dog vessels. J Lab Clin Med 1997;129:356–63.
35. Resta TC, Walker BR, Eichinger MR, et al. Rate of NO scavenging alters effects of recombinant hemoglobin solutions on pulmonary vasoreactivity. J Appl Physiol 2002;93:1327–36.
36. Rudolph AS, Sulpizio A, Hieble P, et al. Liposome encapsulation attenuates hemoglobin-induced vasoconstriction in rabbit arterial segments. J Appl Physiol 1997;82:1826–35.
37. Bone HG, Schenarts PJ, Booke M, et al. Oxalated pyridoxalated hemoglobin polyoxyethylene conjugate normalizes the hyperdynamic circulation in septic sheep. Crit Care Med 1997;25:1010–8.
38. Gulati A, Singh R, Chung SM, et al. Role of endothelin-converting enzyme in the systemic hemodynamics and regional circulatory effects of proendothelin-1 (1–38) and diaspirin cross-linked hemoglobin in rats. J Lab Clin Med 1995;126:559–70.
39. Rohlfs RJ, Bruner E, Chiu A, et al. Arterial blood pressure responses to cell-free hemoglobin solutions and the reaction with nitric oxide. J Biol Chem 1998;273: 12128–34.
40. Sakai H, Hara H, Yuasa M, et al. Molecular dimensions of Hb-based O(2) carriers determine constriction of resistance arteries and hypertension. Am J Physiol Heart Circ Physiol 2000;279:H908–15.
41. Bouwer ST, Hoofd L, Kreuzer F. Diffusion coefficients of oxygen and hemoglobin measured by facilitated oxygen diffusion through hemoglobin solutions. Biochim Biophys Acta 1997;1338:127–36.
42. Nishide H, Chen XS, Tsuchida E. Facilitated oxygen transport with modified and encapsulated hemoglobins across non-flowing solution membrane. Artif Cells Blood Substit Immobil Biotechnol 1997;25:335–46.
43. Lindbom L, Tuma RF, Arfors KE. Influence of oxygen on perfused capillary density and capillary red cell velocity in rabbit skeletal muscle. Microvasc Res 1980;19: 197–208.
44. McCarthy MR, Vandegriff KD, Winslow RM. The role of facilitated diffusion in oxygen transport by cell-free hemoglobins: implications for the design of hemoglobin-based oxygen carriers. Biophys Chem 2001;92:103–17.
45. Winslow RM, Gonzales A, Gonzales ML, et al. Vascular resistance and the efficacy of red cell substitutes in a rat hemorrhage model. J Appl Physiol 1998;85: 993–1003.
46. Wettstein R, Tsai AG, Erni D, et al. Resuscitation with polyethylene glycol-modified human hemoglobin improves microcirculatory blood flow and tissue oxygenation after hemorrhagic shock in awake hamsters. Crit Care Med 2003; 31:1824–30.

47. Gould SA, Moore EE, Hoyt DB, et al. The first randomized trial of human polymerized hemoglobin as a blood substitute in acute trauma and emergent surgery. J Am Coll Surg 1998;187:113–20.
48. Gould SA, Moore EE, Hoyt DB, et al. The life-sustaining capacity of human polymerized hemoglobin when red cells might be unavailable. J Am Coll Surg 2002; 195:445–52.
49. Sloan EP, Koenigsberg M, Gens D, et al. Diaspirin cross-linked hemoglobin (DCLHb) in the treatment of severe traumatic hemorrhagic shock: a randomized controlled efficacy trial. JAMA 1999;282:1857–64.
50. Kerner T, Ahlers O, Veit S, et al. DCL-Hb for trauma patients with severe hemorrhagic shock: the European On-Scene multicenter study. Intensive Care Med 2003;29:378–85.
51. Northfield laboratories reports results of pivotal phase III trauma study [news release]. Evanston (IL): Northfield Laboratories, Inc; 2007. Available at: http://phx.corporate-ir.net/phoenix.zhtml?c=91374&p=irol-newsArticle_print&ID=1005951&highlight=. Accessed June 5, 2008.
52. Schubert A, Przybelski R, Eidt J, et al. Diaspirin-crosslinked haemoglobin reduces blood transfusion in non cardiac surgery: a multicenter, randomized, controlled, double-blinded trial. Anesth Analg 2003;97:323–32.
53. Cheng D, Mazer C, MArtineau R, et al. A phase II dose-response study of hemoglobin raffimer (Hemolink) in elective coronary artery bypass surgery. J Thorac Cardiovasc Surg 2004;127:79–86.
54. Greenburg A, Kim H, Hemolink Study Group. Use of an oxygen therapeutic as an adjunct to intraoperative autologous donation to reduce transfusion requirements in patients undergoing coronary artery bypass surgery. J Am Coll Surg 2004;198: 373–83.
55. Garrioch M, McClure J, Wildsmith J. Haemodynamic effects of diaspirin cross-linked haemoglobin (DCLHb) given before abdominal aortic aneurysm surgery. Br J Anaesth 1999;83:702–7.
56. Bloomfield E, Rady M, Esfandiari S. A prospective trial of diaspirin-linked hemoglobin solution in patients after elective repair of abdominal aortic aneurysm. Mil Med 2004;169:546–50.
57. Olofsson C, Ahl T, Johansson T, et al. A multicenter clinical study of the safety and activity of maleimide-polyethylene glycol-modified Hemoglobin (Hemospan) in patients undergoing major orthopaedic surgery. Anesthesiology 2006;105: 1153–63.
58. Jahr JS, Mackenzie C, Pearce LB, et al. vHBOC-201 as an alternative to blood transfusion: efficacy and safety evaluation in a multicenter phase III trial in elective orthopedic surgery. J Trauma 2008;64:1484–97.
59. Natanson C, Kern S, Lurie P, et al. Cell-free hemoglobin-based blood substitutes and risk of myocardoial infarction and death: a meta-analysis. JAMA 2008;299: 2304–12.
60. Lam C, Tyml K, Martin C, et al. Microvascular perfusion is impaired in a rat model of normotensive sepsis. J Clin Invest 1994;94:2077–83.
61. Sielenkämper AW, Chin-Yee IH, Martin C, et al. Diaspirin crosslinked hemoglobin improves systemic oxygen uptake in oxygen-supply dependent septic rats. Am J Respir Crit Care Med 1997;156:1066–72.
62. Creteur J, Zhang H, De Backer D, et al. Diaspirin cross-linked hemoglobin improves oxygen extraction capabilities in endotoxic shock. J Appl Physiol 2000;89:1437–44.

63. Wong HR, Carcillo JA, Burckart G, et al. Increased serum nitrite and nitrate concentrations in children with the sepsis syndrome. Crit Care Med 1995;23: 835–42.
64. Gomez-Jimenez J, Salgado A, Mourelle M, et al. L-arginine: nitric oxide pathway in endotoxemia and human septic shock. Crit Care Med 1995;23:253–8.
65. Szabo C. Alterations in nitric oxide production in various forms of circulatory shock. New Horiz 1995;3:2–32.
66. Vincent JL, Preiser JC, Zhang H. Blocking the effects of nitric oxide in septic shock. In: Fink MP, Payen D, editors, Role of nitric oxide in septic shock—update in intensive care and emergency medicine, Vol 24. Berlin: Springer-Verlag; 1995. p. 253–73.
67. Lopez A, Lorente JA, Steingrub J, et al. Multiple-center, randomized, double-blind study of the nitric oxide synthase inhibitor 546C88: effect on survival in patients with septic shock. Crit Care Med 2004;32:21–30.
68. Bone HG, Waurick R, Van Aken H, et al. Comparison of the hemodynamic effects of nitric oxide synthase inhibition and nitric oxide scavenging in endotoxemic sheep. Intensive Care Med 1998;24:48–54.
69. Matheson-Urbaitis B, Lu YS, Fronticelli C, et al. Renal and systemic-hemodynamic response to isovolemic exchange transfusion with hemoglobin cross-linked with bis (3, 5-dibromosalicyl) fumarate or albumin. J Lab Clin Med 1995; 126:250–60.
70. Heneka MT, Löschmann PA, Osswald H. Polymerized hemoglobin restores cardiovascular and kidney function in endotoxin-induced shock in the rat. J Clin Invest 1997;99:47–54.
71. Neviere R, Sielenkamper A, Pitt M, et al. Diaspirin crosslinked hemoglobin prevents endotoxin induced myocardial contractile dysfunction in an isolated and perfused rat heart model. Am J Respir Crit Care Med 1997;155:A926 [abstract].
72. Cooper A, Ellis C, Lin HY, et al. Effect of diaspirin crosslinked hemoglobin (DCLHB) treatment on myocardial blood flow heterogeneity in septic sheep. Am J Respir Crit Care Med 1997;155:A926 [abstract].
73. Kinasewitz GT, Imm A, Steingrub JS, et al. Multi-center, randomized, placebo-controlled study of the nitric oxide scavenger pyridoxalated hemoglobin polyoxy-ethylene in distributive shock. Crit Care Med 2008;36:1999–2007.
74. Lee JT, Arenholz DH, Nelson RD, et al. Mechanisms of the adjuvant effect of hemoglobin in experimental peritonitis V: the significance of the coordinated iron component. Surgery 1979;86:41–7.
75. Kim YM, Yamazaki I, Piette LH. The effect of haemoglobin, hematin and iron on neutrophil inactivation in superoxide generating systems. Arch Biochem Biophys 1994;309:308–14.
76. Griffiths E, Cortes A, Gilbert N, et al. Haemoglobin-based blood substitutes and sepsis. Lancet 1995;345:158–60.
77. Su D, Roth RI, Levin J. Hemoglobin infusion augments the tumor necrosis factor response to bacterial endotoxin (lipopolysaccharide) in mice. Crit Care Med 1999;27:771–8.
78. Sherry BA, Alava G, Tracey KJ, et al. Malaria-specific metabolite hemozoin mediates the release of several potent endogenous pyrogens (TNF, MIP-1α and MIP-1β) in vitro, and altered thermoregulation in vivo. J Inflamm 1995;45:85–96.
79. McFaul SJ, Bowman PD, Villa VM, et al. Hemoglobin stimulates mononuclear cells to release interleukin-8 and tumor necrosis factor α. Blood 1994;84:3175–81.

80. Carrillo EH, Gordon LE, Richardson JD, et al. Free hemoglobin enhances tumor necrosis factor-alpha production in isolated human monocytes. J Trauma 2002; 52:449–52.
81. Rabinovici R, Rudolph AS, Vernick J, et al. Lyophilized liposome encapsulated hemoglobin: evaluation of hemodynamic, biochemical, and hematologic responses. Crit Care Med 1994;22:480–5.
82. Rudolph AS, Cliff R, Kwasiborski V, et al. Liposome-encapsulated hemoglobin modulates lipopolysaccharide-induced tumor necrosis factor-α production in mice. Crit Care Med 1997;25:460–8.
83. Chappell JE, McBride WJ, Shackford SR. Diaspirin cross-linked hemoglobin resuscitation improves cerebral perfusion after head injury and shock. J Trauma 1996;41:781–8.
84. Bowes MP, Burhop KE, Zivin JA. Diaspirin cross-linked hemoglobin improves neurological outcome following reversible but not irreversible CNS ischemia in rabbits. Stroke 1994;25:2253–7.
85. Cole DJ, Schell RM, Drummond JC, et al. Focal cerebral ischemia in rats: effect of hemodilution with α-α cross-linked hemoglobin on brain injury. Can J Neurol Sci 1993;20:30–6.
86. Saxena R, Wijnhoud AD, Carton H, et al. Controlled safety study of a hemoglobin-based oxygen carrier, DCLHb, in acute ischemic stroke. Stroke 1999;30:993–6.
87. George I, Yi G, Schulman A, et al. A polymerized bovine haemoglobin oxygen carrier preserves regional myocardial function and reduces infarct size after acute myocardial ischemia. Am J Physiol Heart Circ Physiol 2006;291:H1126–37.
88. Burmeister M, Rempf C, Standl T, et al. Effect of prophylactic or therapeutic application of bovine haemoglobin HBOC-200 on ischaemia-reperfusion injury following acute coronary ligature in rats. Br J Anaesth 2005;95:737–45.
89. Caswell J, Strange M, Rimmer D, et al. A novel hemoglobin-based blood substitute protects against myocardial reperfusion injury. Am J Physiol Heart Circ Physiol 2005;288:H1796–801.
90. Raff JP, Dobson CE, Tsai H. Transfusion of polymerized human haemoglobin in a patient with severe sickle-cell anaemia. Lancet 2002;60:464–5.
91. Lanzkron S, Moliterno AR, Norris EJ, et al. Polymerized human Hb use in acute chest syndrome: a case report. Transfusion 2002;42:1422–6.
92. Gonzalez P, Hackney AC, Jones S, et al. A phase I/II study of polymerized bovine hemoglobin in adult patients with sickle. J Investig Med 1997;45:258–64.

The USA Multicenter Prehosptial Hemoglobin-based Oxygen Carrier Resuscitation Trial: Scientific Rationale, Study Design, and Results

Ernest E. Moore, MD[a],*, Jeffrey L. Johnson, MD[a],
Frederick A. Moore, MD[b], Hunter B. Moore, BA[c]

KEYWORDS

- Hemoglobin-based oxygen carrier • Blood substitute
- Prehospital resuscitation • Hemorrhagic shock • Trauma

The current generation of blood substitutes tested in clinical trials are red blood cell (RBC) substitutes; that is, they are designed primarily to transport oxygen. The products now being used in advanced-phase clinical trials are derived from hemoglobin (Hb) and are thus often referred to as Hb-based oxygen carriers (HBOCs). The potential benefits of HBOCs are well known (**Box 1**). The objectives of this overview are to provide the scientific background and rationale for the study design of the USA Multicenter Prehospital HBOC Resuscitation Trial and to present the results and discuss clinical implications.

This article has contains data from the following references: **26–28, 45, 47–49, 52, 59, and 74.**
Supported in part by Northfield Laboratories, Inc. and National Institutes of Health Grants P50GM49222, T32GM08315, and U54GM62119.
[a] Department of Surgery, Denver Health Medical Center, University of Colorado Health Sciences Center, 777 Bannock Street, Denver, CO 80204, USA
[b] Department of Surgery, Methodist Hospital and Weill-Cornell University, Houston, TX, USA
[c] University of Vermont School of Medicine, Burlington, VT, USA
* Corresponding author.
E-mail address: ernest.moore@dhha.org (E.E. Moore).

Box 1
Potential clinical benefits of hemoglobin-based oxygen carriers in trauma care

Availability

Abundant supply

Universally compatible

Prolonged shelf-life

Storage at room temperature

Safety

No disease transmissions

No antigenic reactions

No immunologic effects

Efficacy

Enhanced oxygen delivery

Improved rheologic properties

POTENTIAL ROLE OF HEMOGLOBIN-BASED OXYGEN CARRIERS IN TRAUMA CARE

The US Food and Drug Administration (FDA) approval of a new product proceeds through phase I, II, and III studies designed to establish safety and efficacy (**Table 1**). FDA regulation defines efficacy as follows: "Effectiveness means a reasonable expectation that...the pharmacologic or other effect of the biologic product...will serve a clinically significant function in the diagnosis, cure, mitigation, treatment, or prevention of disease in man."[1] The Center for Biologics Evaluation and Research (CBER) is the review body for the FDA in the arena of biologies and has published a comprehensive listing of "points to consider in the safety evaluation of HBOCs."[2]

Table 1
Potential role of hemoglobin-based oxygen carriers in trauma care

Application	Location
Perioperative applications	
Reduce allogeneic RBC transfusions	ED, angiography, OR, ICU
Attenuate transfusion immunodulation	OR, ICU
Acute hemorrhagic shock	
When stored RBCs are unavailable	Field, ED, OR, ICU, remote hospital, civilian disaster, military conflict
More efficient resuscitation	Field, ED, OR, ICU
Low-volume resuscitation	Remote hospital, civilian disaster, military conflict
Regional perfusion	
Enhance oxygen delivery	
Ischemic reperfusion tissue/organ	OR, ICU
Inflamed tissue	OR, ICU
Ex vivo organ perfusion	Hospital, OR

Abbreviations: ED, Emergency department; OR, Operating room.

These points encompass characterization of the product, animal safety testing, and human studies and address the theoretic concerns of Hb solutions raised previously,[3–6] including pulmonary and systemic hypertension, organ dysfunction, oxidative tissue injury, synergy with bacterial pathogens, and immunomodulation. In 1994, CBER convened a workshop with the National Heart, Lung, and Blood Institute and the Department of the Army to develop "points to consider in the efficacy evaluation of HBOCs."[7] Documenting a direct clinical end point for HBOCs is challenging because this end point has never been established for RBCs. Specific recommendations for clinical studies are in three areas: perioperative applications, acute hemorrhagic shock, and regional perfusion. Field trials for postinjury hemorrhagic shock, where RBCs are not available, are difficult because of safety and ethical issues. Decreased perioperative allogeneic RBC transfusion is regarded as a clinical benefit, but the potential risks of HBOCs also need to be defined and evaluated. Regional perfusion studies include reperfusion following ischemia (eg, as an adjunct during coronary angioplasty; the FDA approved Fluosol DA in 1989 as an oxygen-carrying drug for this setting).

CLINICAL EVALUATION OF MODIFIED TETRAMERIC HEMOGLOBIN IN TRAUMA CARE: THE FIRST MULTICENTER TRIAL

Of the modified Hb tetrameric solutions that looked promising in the late 1980s, one formulation was authorized by the FDA for a phase III study in trauma. HemAssist (Baxter, Boulder, Colorado) consisted of Hb tetramers cross-linked between α subunits with bis 3,5 diabromosalicyl fumarate to prevent dissociation into dimers and to reduce oxygen affinity. It is unfortunate that this clinical trial failed.[8] Regarded by some as a major setback for HBOCs, it is important to emphasize that this United States multicenter trial of diaspirin cross-linked Hb (DCLHb) for the treatment of severe traumatic hemorrhagic shock was based on the explicit proposal that "DCLHb was tested not as a substitute for blood but rather as an adjunct to the currently used therapies for enhancing oxygen delivery: fluids, blood, and operative intervention." Although the unexpected outcome raised the issue of comparable study groups, the difference in the primary study end point was concerning: the 28-day mortality for the DCLHb group was 46% (24/52) compared with 17% (8/46) for the control (normal saline) group. Much expert thought and preparation went into the study design of this human trial, but the scientific justification of using a vasoconstricting agent for the initial resuscitation of acute hemorrhagic shock was, in retrospect, questionable.

The investigators rationalized this study design because in preclinical trials, "DCLHb has been shown to be effective in enhancing perfusion in small volumes, suggesting a pharmacologic effect that is independent of hemoglobin." The pharmacologic effect, however, was not always reported as beneficial. In 1993, Hess and coauthors,[9] at the Letterman Army Institute of Research, reported that in a swine model of hemorrhagic shock, DCLHb infusion doubled systemic and pulmonary vascular resistance and that these responses were associated with a fall in cardiac output. In fact, these changes were equivalent to resuscitation with unmodified tetrameric Hb. Hess and colleagues[9] concluded, "the decrease in cardiac output associated with the vasoconstriction in the Hb-treated animals was equal to the increase in oxygen-carrying capacity—crystalloid or colloid solutions provided equally rapid correction of the elevated whole blood lactate." In a follow-up study,[10] the infusion of low-dose (4 mL/kg = 14 g Hb) DCLHb into swine subjected to hemorrhagic shock prompted the investigators to further warn "pulmonary hypertension and low peripheral perfusion may offset benefits for trauma patients." Although the DCLHb trial investigators cited several animal models that appeared to support their study hypothesis, none of these models replicated their study design—a lesson for the future conduct of clinical trials with HBOCs.

The mechanisms responsible for the vasoconstriction resulting from DCLHb administration were investigated before the trauma clinical trial. The increased vascular resistance was believed to be mediated predominantly by the scavenging of nitric oxide (NO), with an additional component of enhanced endothelin release.[11–13] Subsequently, alternative mechanisms were proposed, including release-enhanced adrenergic receptor sensitivity and reduced arterial wall shear stress secondary to decreased viscosity.[14,15] Development of DCLHb has been terminated, but the relevance of these basic mechanisms to future trauma care with HBOCs is clear.

CLINICAL SAFETY OF POLYMERIZED HEMOGLOBIN IN TRAUMA CARE

At this moment, the HBOCs currently tested in phase III trials are polymerized Hb solutions (**Table 2**). Polymerization addresses several of the problems inherent in tetrameric Hb: short intravascular retention and reduced colloid osmotic activity. Polymerization also appears to attenuate vasoconstriction associated with the infusion of Hb solutions. A proposed explanation is that tetrameric Hb (65 kd) extravasates through the endothelium to bind abluminal NO, leading to unopposed vasoconstriction, whereas polymerized Hb (>130 kd) remains in the vasculature to bind only luminal NO. Of interest, Hb of the common earthworm, Lumbricus terrestris, is a polymer with a molecular weight of 400 kd that circulates extracellularly.[16] Mice and rats undergoing exchange transfusion with this naturally occurring polymeric Hb showed no changes in behavior, and nuclear magnetic resonance spectroscopy of the heart confirmed normal oxygen-carrying capacity.[17]

Polymerized HBOCs have undergone extensive preclinical and clinical testing for safety. Hemopure (Biopure Corp, Cambridge, Massachusetts), a polymer of bovine Hb, has been used successfully to reduce allogeneic RBC transfusion in elective cardiac,[18] aortic,[19] and hepatic[20] surgery. One study with abdominal aortic reconstruction raised concern about increased systemic vascular resistance,[21] an effect identified in normal volunteers.[22] Recent animal studies designed to replicate prehospital

Table 2
Characteristics of current hemoglobin-based oxygen carriers in phase III trials

Characteristic	Hemopure	PolyHeme	RBCs
Hemoglobin (g%)	13	10	13
Unit equivalent (g)	30	50	50
Molecular weight (>64 kd)	≥95%	≥99%	≥100%
P_{50} (mm Hg)	38	29	26
Hill coefficient	1.4	1.7	2.7
Oncotic pressure (mm Hg)	25	23	25
Viscosity (cp)	1.3	2.1	(Whole blood 5–10)
Methemoglobin (%)	<10	<8	<1
Half-life	19 h	24 h	31 d
Shelf-life at 4°C	≥3 y	≥1.5 y	42 d
Shelf-life at 21°C	≥2 y	≥6 wk	≥6 h

Abbreviations: cp, Centipoise; P_{50}, Tension when hemoglobin-binding sites are 50% saturated.

hypotensive resuscitation for hemorrhagic shock have been encouraging.[23–25] Hemopure has been approved for replacement of acute blood loss in South Africa, but there are no published results to date. PolyHeme (Northfield Laboratories, Evanston, Illinois) has been evaluated predominantly in acutely injured patients. PolyHeme is derived from outdated human stored blood. After lysis of RBCs, the native tetrameric Hb is polymerized with glutaraldehyde. Pyridoxal phosphate is used to obtain a more physiologic P_{50}. The meticulous, multistep biochemical purification of PolyHeme is believed to eliminate the risk of infection transmission. Under FDA guidance, the authors initiated clinical trials in trauma to confirm safety with escalating doses of PolyHeme. In the first clinical trail,[26] 39 patients received one (n = 14), two (n = 2), three (n = 15), or six (n = 8) units of PolyHeme as their initial resuscitation after acute blood loss. Infusion rates ranged from one unit in 175 minutes to six units (300 g) in 20 minutes. Although the RBC Hb fell to 2.9 ± 0.2 g%, total Hb was maintained at 7.5 ± 0.2 g% with PolyHeme. With respect to safety, the patient's temperature, mean arterial pressure, heart rate, and creatinine clearance did not change during the 72-hour study period. Liver function tests and amylase varied substantially because of patient injuries. Cognizant of the vasoconstriction associated with the DCLHb clinical trial, the authors designed a study to specifically evaluate the vascular response to PolyHeme infusion in acutely injured patients.[27] Patients requiring urgent transfusion were administered PolyHeme (up to six units) or stored RBCs during their initial resuscitation. Systemic arterial pressure, pulmonary arterial pressure, cardiac index, and pulmonary capillary wedge pressure were measured every 4 hours post infusion. There were no significant differences between the groups for these indices or the calculated systemic or pulmonary vascular resistance. Additional issues reported with the clinical use of polymerized Hb solutions included interference of laboratory tests that are based on colormetric changes from dissolved plasma Hb, inaccuracy of oxygen saturation monitoring because of methemoglobin, mild elevations of serum amylase (but without evidence of pancreatitis), and skin rashes. None of these issues has been considered a clinically significant adverse event to date.

CLINICAL EFFICACY OF POLYMERIZED HEMOGLOBIN IN TRAUMA CARE
Perioperative Applications: Reduce Allogeneic Red Blood Cell Transfusions in Trauma Care

Prompted by the FDA guidelines to demonstrate efficacy, all HBOC companies pursued what appeared to be the simplest clinically: to reduce the need for allogeneic RBC transfusions. In collaboration with David B. Hoyt, MD, and the University of California at San Diego, the authors conducted a randomized trial in patients requiring urgent transfusion.[28] The 44 trauma patients (injury severity score [ISS] = 21 ± 1.3) were allocated to receive stored RBCs or up to six units of PolyHeme as their initial blood replacement. The RBC Hb was equivalent preinfusion (10.4 ± 0.4 g% versus 9.4 ± 0.3 g%); at end infusion, the RBC Hb of the PolyHeme patients fell to 5.8 ± 0.5 g% versus 10.6 ± 0.3 g% in the control subjects. The PolyHeme group received 4.4 ± 0.3 units, resulting in a plasma Hb of 3.9 ± 0.2 g%. The total number of allogeneic RBC transfusions for the control group compared with the PolyHeme group was 10.4 ± 0.9 units versus 6.8 ± 0.9 units ($P<.05$) through day 1, and 11.3 ± 0.9 units versus 7.8 ± 0.9 units ($P = .06$) through day 3. After the initial phase, infusion of 4.6 units of stored RBCs in the control group was equivalent to the 5.2 units in the PolyHeme group. Both volumes presumably represented the infused RBCs or PolyHeme lost during acute hemorrhage before operative control. Subsequent replacement volumes were comparable, ultimately sparing the PolyHeme group approximately four units of allogeneic RBC transfusion.

Perioperative Applications: Reduce Allogenic Red Blood Cell Transfusions During Initial Resuscitation and Thereby Decrease Acute Respiratory Distress Syndrome and Multiple Organ Failure

With the authors' long-term interest in the pathogenesis of postinjury multiple organ failure (MOF),[29,30] their working hypothesis extended beyond reduced stored blood use during hospitalization. The authors proposed that PolyHeme, in lieu of stored RBCs during initial resuscitation, would attenuate the adverse immunoinflammatory effects of allogeneic RBC transfusion and ultimately reduce the incidence of acute respiratory distress syndrome (ARDS) and MOF. Stored blood is reportedly safer than ever due to comprehensive screening for disease transmission, but the potential adverse effects of packed RBC storage on the immune response to injury and illness are becoming more apparent.[31,32] The authors have been interested in the proinflammatory effects of stored RBCs and specifically in their capacity to provoke polymorphonuclear neutrophil (PMN) cytotoxicity. The PMN is a key cellular mediator in the pathogenesis of postinjury MOF. Consequently, PMN functional responses are evaluated as a clinical surrogate for the two-event model of MOF: inflammatory priming and subsequent activation. The two-event construct of postinjury MOF is based on the fundamental concept that injury primes the innate immune system such that a second insult, during this vulnerable window, provokes unbridled systemic inflammation, resulting in organ dysfunction.[33] Priming is defined as an enhanced response to a stimulus that is due to prior exposure of the cell to a different agonist.[34] In the authors' ongoing epidemiologic studies,[35] they have shown that more than six units of RBC transfusion within the first 12 hours post injury is an independent risk factor for MOF.[36] Furthermore, the age of the transfused blood within the first 6 hours post injury correlates with the incidence of MOF.[37] Previous studies in the authors' center have shown that after severe injury, patients at high risk for MOF have circulating PMNs that are primed for cytotoxicity within the first 6 hours post injury, as marked by the increased surface expression CD11b/CD18, p 38 mitogen-activated protein kinase activation, release of cytotoxic products in response to formyl-methionyl-leucyl-phenylalanine, and delayed apoptosis.[38]

The precise mechanisms linking packed RBC transfusion and PMN priming remain to be established, but many believe that passenger leukocytes accompanying RBCs in storage are important in the generation of proinflammatory agents.[39] Plasma from stored RBCs primes PMNs in vitro, and this effect has been shown to increase progressively from 14 to 42 days of storage.[40] Some investigators have incriminated cytokines (tumor necrosis factor α, interleukin [IL]-1, IL-6, IL-8, and IL-18) generated during storage,[41] whereas the authors have focused on proinflammatory lipids leukotriene β_4 and lysophosphatidylcholine) presumably generated from the RBC membrane.[42] Metabolites of the arachidonic acid cascade have been strongly implicated in the pathogenesis of transfusion-related acute lung injury.[43] Although prestorage leukoreduction of RBCs decreases the generation of cytokines, this process does not eliminate PMN priming.[44] Thus, collectively, these studies suggest that a blood substitute devoid of proinflammatory agents will avoid the immunomodulatory consequences of allogeneic RBCs.

In preparation for clinical trials, the authors conducted in vitro and in vivo studies to test their hypothesis that PolyHeme—free of inflammatory cytokines and lipids—would eliminate the PMN priming previously documented with stored RBCs and translate to reduced ARDS and MOF.[45] Human PMNs were isolated from healthy volunteers, and the plasma fraction was separated from packed RBCs at 42 days of storage in the authors' blood bank (day 42 is the last day that stored RBCs can be transfused clinically, but often, these are the first RBCs infused into trauma patients).[46]

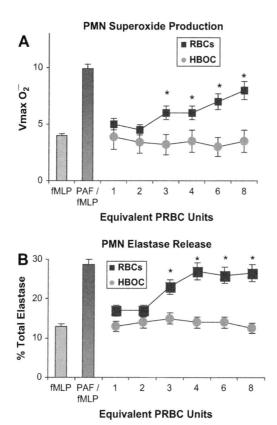

Fig. 1. Isolated human neutrophils (PMNs) were incubated with the plasma fraction from stored RBCs or PolyHeme at concentrations equivalent to one through eight units of acute transfusion. (*A*) PMN superoxide production. (*B*) PMN elastase release. Formyl-methionyl-leucyl-phenylalanine (fMLP) is employed as a PMN activator, and platelet-activating factor (PAF; primer) followed by fMLP approximates maximal PMN response. *$P<.05$.

The isolated PMNs were incubated with RBC plasma or PolyHeme at concentrations calculated to be equivalent up to eights units of transfusion. The plasma fraction representing three or more units of stored RBCs primed the human PMNs for enhanced superoxide production and elastase release (**Fig. 1**).

The authors further tested their hypothesis in an established two-event model of MOF: trauma/hemorrhagic shock as a priming event followed by toll-like receptor 4 engagement as an activating event.[47] The primary study objective was to contrast HBOCs versus crystalloid in the prehospital phase, but the study groups were expanded to encompass the possible availability of stored blood in the field and the authors' previous in-hospital phase II clinical work with HBOC resuscitation. Acute lung injury was selected as the primary study end point because ARDS is the first manifestation of postinjury MOF. Rats underwent laparotomy and hemorrhagic shock (30 mm Hg × 45 minutes) and were resuscitated over 2 hours in a clinically relevant design: two times the volume of shed blood (SB) using normal saline in the first 30 minutes; one half the volume of SB in the next 30 minutes; another two times SB volume with normal saline over the remaining 60 minutes. Four study groups represented alternative fluid strategies during the first hour of resuscitation: in-hospital SB (standard resuscitation); in-hospital HBOC; prehospital SB; and prehospital HBOC. Global physiologic response was assessed by way of tissue oxygenation (near infrared spectroscopy) and arterial base deficit; pulmonary response was assessed by way of lung neutrophil (PMN) accumulation and vascular permeability. Prehospital HBOC resuscitation provided the most efficient recovery of tissue oxygenation (**Fig. 2**) and correction of base deficit, had the greatest reduction in pulmonary PMN accumulation, and abrogated acute lung injury (**Fig. 3**). The findings in this controlled in vivo study further supported the authors' hypothesis that initial HBOC resuscitation attenuates the postshock inflammatory response and secondary organ dysfunction.

In the authors' subsequent clinical trial, injured patients requiring urgent transfusion were administered PolyHeme (up to 20 units = 1000 g) or stored RBCs for their initial 12 hours of resuscitation.[48] PMN priming was determined by the surface expression of CD11b/CD18 in whole blood and by superoxide production in isolated PMNs. The study groups (stored RBCs [n = 10] versus PolyHeme [n = 9]) were comparable with respect to injury severity (ISS: 27.9 ± 4.5 versus 21.9 ± 2.7), physiologic compromise (emergency department pH: 7.22 ± 0.04 versus 7.19 ± 0.08), and Hb transfusion in the first 24 hours (units: 14.1 ± 2.0 versus 14.5 ± 1). Circulating PMNs from patients resuscitated with stored RBCs manifested evidence of priming through increased CD11b/CD18 expression and enhanced superoxide production (**Fig. 4**). Three patients (30%) in the stored RBC group died of MOF, whereas all patients in the PolyHeme group survived.

To further investigate the impact of early resuscitation with PolyHeme in lieu of stored RBCs, the authors extended the clinical trial to evaluate the systemic levels of proinflammatory cytokines (IL-6, IL-8), counterregulatory cytokines (IL-10, IL-11), and markers of endothelial activation (sICAM, sE-selectin).[49] The study groups (stored RBCs [n = 7] versus PolyHeme [n = 18]) were comparable with respect to injury severity. Patients resuscitated with stored RBCs had higher levels of the proinflammatory cytokines IL-6 and IL-8 and higher levels of the counterregulatory cytokine IL-10 (**Fig. 5**), with a trend toward higher sICAM and sE-selectin levels. The authors did not

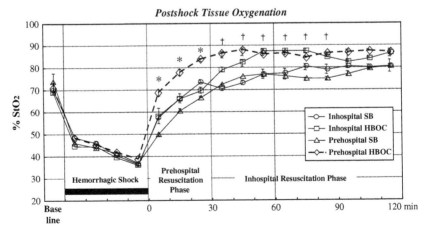

Fig. 2. Tissue oxygenation (StO2 = tissue oxygen saturation) was monitored continuously with a near infrared spectroscopy device placed on the animal's hind limb. Prehospital HBOC and Inhospital HBOC versus Prehospital SB and Inhospital SB, *$P<.05$ versus other groups; $^{\dagger}P<.05$.

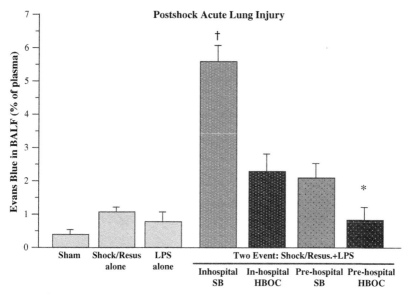

Fig. 3. Acute lung injury, determined by Evans blue alveolar extravasation, was evaluated at the end of the study (8 hours post insult). Simulated prehospital HBOC resuscitated abrogated early acute lung injury. *$P<.05$ versus Inhospital SB; †$P<.05$ versus all other Two-Event groups. BALF, bronchoalveolar lavage fluid; LPS, lipopolysaccharide; Resus, resuscitated.

enroll a sufficient number of injured patients to definitively address the ultimate study objective—reduction of postinjury MOF; however, the incidence of MOF in the acutely injured patients given PolyHeme during their initial resuscitation for whom the authors had complete data (n = 20) was 15%, contrasted with a predicted incidence of 37% ($P<.05$) based on their MOF prediction model.[45] In sum, these clinical trials in trauma patients suggest that PolyHeme, used in the early resuscitation of patients who have hemorrhagic shock, attenuates the immunodysfunction associated with stored RBC transfusion and thereby reduces the incidence of postinjury MOF.

Acute Hemorrhagic Shock: When Stored Red Blood Cells are Unavailable in Trauma Care

The most compelling indication for HBOC is the scenario in which stored RBCs are unavailable. This potential benefit for military use has largely driven the development of HBOCs, but there are also a number of key applications in civilian trauma care. Most conspicuous is the role in prehospital care, particularly for extended transport times, but there are also remote hospitals throughout the country in which stored blood is simply not available or is rapidly depleted when multiple casualties are encountered. Well-designed animal models have strongly suggested that prehospital low-volume resuscitation with HBOCs can save lives.[23–25]

Despite the evidence, the scientific design and ethical conduct of clinical trials to establish efficacy of HBOCs when RBCs are unavailable remain a challenge.[50,51] To best approximate this scenario, the authors compared the 30-day mortality in 171 trauma patients given up to 20 units (1000 g) of PolyHeme with a historic control group of 300 surgical patients who refused stored RBCs on religious grounds.[52] The trauma patients received rapid infusion of 1 to 2 units (n = 45), 3 to 4 units (n = 45), 5 to 9 units (n = 47), or 10 to 20 units (n = 34) of PolyHeme; 40 patients had a nadir RBC Hb of 3

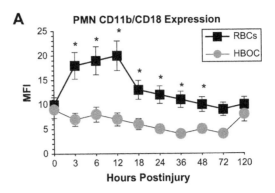

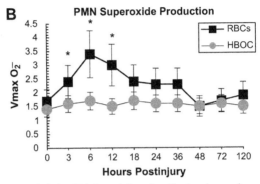

Fig. 4. Circulating neutrophils (PMNs) from injured patients who underwent initial resuscitation with stored RBCs or PolyHeme. (*A*) PMN CD11b/CD18 receptor expression in whole blood. (*B*) PMN superoxide production in isolated cells. *$P<.05$.

g% or less (mean 1.5 ± 0.7 g%). Total Hb was adequately maintained (mean 6.8 ± 1.2 g%) by way of plasma Hb added by PolyHeme. The 30-day mortality was 25.0% (10/40) in the PolyHeme group compared with 64.5% (20/31) in the control group (**Fig. 6**).

A personal experience with PolyHeme during the authors' in-hospital FDA-approved phase II studies convinced them that the time had arrived for licensing of HBOCs for trauma care.[45] An 18-year-old man arrived by ground ambulance at the emergency department in extremis after a gunshot wound to the abdomen from a high-velocity elk-hunting rifle (30.06, hollow soft-point 220 gr, muzzle energy 2840 ft/lb). Because of immediate availability, 10 units of PolyHeme (maximal dose permitted at that time) were administered during the first 14 minutes of in-hospital resuscitation, representing greater than 91% of total circulating Hb at end infusion (RBC Hb = 0.7 g%). The missile entered the left midabdomen and exited posteriorly. At laparotomy, the authors encountered an avulsed shattered left kidney with secondary aortic and vena caval perforations, a partially transected superior mesenteric vein, and destructive injuries to the patient's distal duodenum, proximal jejunum, midileum, and descending and sigmoid colon. In addition, the patient had massive soft tissue loss in the retroperitoneum, including the psoas and paraspinous muscles, and suffered a concussive spinal cord lesion with resultant paraplegia. The patient received an additional 40 units of packed RBCs during initial laparotomy but, ultimately, this man survived to discharge without organ failure. The authors believe that the immediate infusion of this HBOC was pivotal in maintaining sufficient oxygen delivery during the critical period of massive blood loss to help save this man's life.

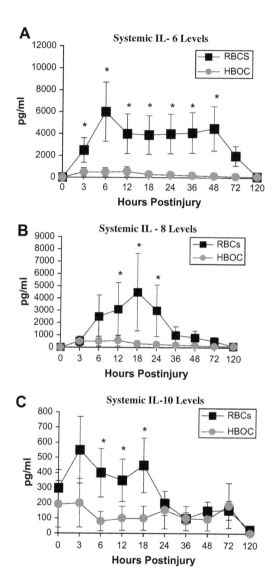

Fig. 5. Systemic IL-6 (*A*), IL-8 (*B*), and IL-10 (*C*) from injured patients who underwent initial resuscitation with stored RBCs or PolyHeme. *$P<.05$.

PHASE III USA MULTICENTER PREHOSPITAL HBOC RESUSCITATION TRIAL

The optimal resuscitation fluid for acute blood loss remains unclear, and the practical options for prehospital care have been limited to expansion of the circulating blood volume. The issue is magnified in the combat scenario in which access to blood transfusion is further delayed.[53] Resurgent interest in defining optimal field resuscitation has challenged the long-standing practice of unbridled crystalloid loading,[54] citing the potential risk of exacerbating hemorrhage by way of dislodging hemostatic clots[55] and diluting plasma coagulation factors. Conversely, the magnitude of oxygen debt following hemorrhagic shock correlates directly with adverse outcome.[56–58] The availability of HBOCs offers a new strategy for this clinical "catch 22." Consequently, with

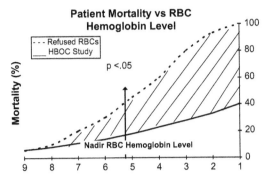

Fig. 6. Comparison of 30-day mortality in surgical patients who refused stored RBC transfusion versus injured patients who were initially resuscitated with PolyHeme. Computer-generated curves are based on nadir Hb levels. Mortality was significantly less (*P*<.05) in the PolyHeme group when RBC Hb was 5.3 g% or less (critical anemia).

this background and preliminary data, the authors conducted a multicenter prehospital trial in the United States.[59]

The objective of this trial was to assess survival of patients in hemorrhagic shock by comparing treatments initiated at the scene: PolyHeme versus standard of care (crystalloid in the field followed by stored RBCs at hospital arrival). The protocol was based on two potential survival benefits: (1) early replacement of oxygen-carrying capacity in a setting where blood is unavailable, and (2) the use of PolyHeme in lieu of allogeneic RBCs during the first 12 hours post injury to reduce the immunoinflammatory response and subsequent organ dysfunction.

Study Design

In this controlled, open-label trial, patients were randomized in the prehospital setting to the PolyHeme group or the control group (Control). The inclusion criteria were presumed acute blood loss from trauma, class III hemorrhagic shock (systolic blood pressure [SBP] ≤90 mm Hg), and age 18 years or older. Exclusion criteria included imminent death, cardiopulmonary resuscitation, severe head injury (Glasgow Coma Scale [GCS] ≤5), pregnancy, or religious objection to blood products. Patient enrollment occurred under FDA regulation 21CFR§50.24 (**Box 2**), providing for exception from informed consent.[60] Study sites were level I trauma centers. The study design is outlined in **Fig. 7**. PolyHeme patients received up to six units (50 g Hb/unit) of PolyHeme beginning at the scene of injury and during the first 12 hours post injury. If needed, stored RBCs were given thereafter. Control patients received crystalloid in the field and stored RBCs as needed in the hospital. Transfusion triggers were based on recent National Institutes of Health Glue Grant protocols for the resuscitation of hemorrhagic shock.[61]

Study End Points

The primary efficacy end point was day 30 mortality. Secondary efficacy end points were day 30 mortality for injury-type subgroups (blunt versus penetrating), day 1 mortality, allogeneic blood use through day 1, and the incidence of MOF through day 30. MOF scores were calculated using the Denver MOF score,[36] which evaluated four organ systems (lung, kidney, liver, and heart), each graded zero to three with an MOF threshold of four or greater after 48 hours post injury. Primary and secondary safety end points included day 1 mortality, day 30 mortality, adverse events (AEs), and serious AEs (SAEs).

Box 2
Exception from informed consent requirements for emergency research in the United States

Human subjects are in a life-threatening situation; available treatments are unsatisfactory.

Obtaining informed consent is not feasible.

Participation in the research holds out the prospect of direct benefit to the subjects.

The clinical investigation could not practicably be performed without the waiver.

The investigational plan defines the length of the potential therapeutic window; the investigator has committed to attempting to contact a legally authorized representative during that window.

Statistical Analysis

The primary efficacy analysis was a dual superiority/noninferiority assessment of day 30 mortality.[62–67] The study design assumed a mortality rate of 17% for the control group based on published series.[8,54,68,69] The superiority hypothesis assumed that PolyHeme patients would have a 7% lower mortality rate compared with Control patients. The superiority outcome was based on the potential benefit of (1) providing an oxygen carrier during prehospital critical anemia, and (2) avoiding allogeneic blood transfusion–related MOF in the first 12 hours. The noninferiority hypothesis assumed that PolyHeme patients would have no more than a 7% higher mortality rate compared with Control patients. Different noninferiority margins were considered, but 7% was chosen based on available medical literature, the feasibility of the study, earlier work in acute blood loss patients compared with historical control subjects,[52] and a study of injured and bleeding patients who were administered blood en route to the medical center.[70] The implication of a noninferiority outcome is that PolyHeme would not be used interchangeably with available RBCs. Rather, in contrast with traditional noninferiority trials, a noninferiority outcome in this trial would allow the benefit to be extrapolated to settings in which RBCs are needed but not available.

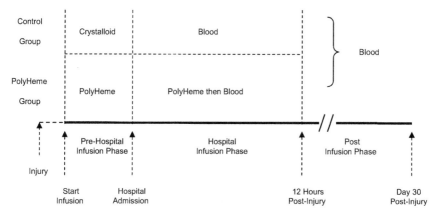

Fig. 7. Study design. Patients were randomized (50:50) into each treatment group. PolyHeme patients received PolyHeme in the field, then PolyHeme (up to six units) for up to 12 hours, and then blood in the hospital, as needed. Control patients received crystalloid in the field, then RBC transfusion in the hospital as needed. (*Adapted from* Moore EE, Moore FA, Fabian TC, et al. Human polymerized hemoglobin for the treatment of hemorrhagic shock when blood is unavailable: the USA Multicenter Trial. J Am Coll Surg 2009;208:1–13; with permission.)

Using a one-sided 0.05 alpha level, the study was powered for both hypotheses at 720 patients. An independent data monitoring committee (IDMC) comprising three experts in trauma, critical care, and biostatistics convened following enrollment of 60, 120, 250, and 500 patients to perform blinded safety analyses. A blinded adaptive power analysis was performed after enrollment of 250 patients to ensure that no increase in the trial size was necessary. In the final analysis, the confidence interval on the difference between mortalities was used in a nonparametric analysis of covariance,[62–67] adjusting for the following covariates: age, sex, mechanism of injury, ISS, GCS, field SBP, and amount of prerandomization crystalloid. The alpha level was adjusted to correct for the IDMC interim analyses.

Results

Enrollment occurred from January 2004 to July 2006 at 29 level I trauma centers. Demographics and baseline characteristics were comparable between groups (**Table 3**), with the exception of coagulation status. Within the 12-hour postinjury interval, 53% of patients in the PolyHeme group received one to two units, 15% received three to five units, and 32% received six units. Of the Control patients, 7% received one to two units of RBCs, 10% received three to five units, and 34% received at least six units in the initial 12-hour postinjury interval. At 6 and 12 hours post injury, PolyHeme patients had a mean [Hb] of 10.4 g/dL and 10.3 g/dL, respectively; Control patients had a mean [Hb] of 11.2 g/dL and 10.8 g/dL, respectively.

Cohort Analyses

Three prespecified cohorts were analyzed (**Fig. 8**). Six of the 720 patients received no study treatment. The primary efficacy analysis was based on the remaining 714 patients analyzed according to the treatment to which they were randomized ("As Randomized"). Safety was analyzed in the 714 patients based on the treatment actually received ("As Treated"). The "Per Protocol" cohort included 590 randomized patients who did not violate predefined major eligibility or treatment regimen criteria. There were 124 (17%) patients who had major protocol violations (71 PolyHeme, 53 Control).

Primary Efficacy End Point

Day 30 mortality rates and confidence intervals for the three cohorts and the "Major Protocol Violations" group are shown in **Table 4** and **Fig. 9**. There was no significant difference in mortality between the PolyHeme and Control groups. The upper limit of the confidence interval exceeded the 7% noninferiority threshold in the As Randomized (7.65%) and the As Treated cohorts (7.06%). In the Per Protocol cohort, the upper limit of the confidence interval was below the 7% threshold (6.21%).

Following the day 30 assessment, four patient deaths in the As Randomized cohort were reported. One patient died on day 32 who was randomized to Control and received PolyHeme. A second patient died on day 34 who was randomized to and received Control. A third patient died on day 41 who was randomized to and received Control. A fourth patient died on day 194 who was randomized to and received PolyHeme. Two additional patients died (one PolyHeme and one Control) who were randomized but did not receive any treatment with study fluids (saline, PolyHeme, or RBCs).

Secondary Efficacy End Points

Day 1 mortality was not significantly different between PolyHeme and Control in any cohort (As Randomized: 35/350 [10.0%] versus 27/364 [7.4%]; As Treated: 34/349

[9.7%] versus 28/365 [7.7%]; Per Protocol: 20/279 [7.2%] versus 22/311 [7.1%]). This end point is an important one because day 1 represents a clinically relevant prolonged interval of delayed access to RBCs. The administration of PolyHeme, up to six units in the first 12 hours, simulated such a delay in access to stored RBCs.

Blunt deaths were statistically higher in the PolyHeme group, but there was no treatment-by-covariate interaction for mechanism of injury in any cohort (see **Table 4**). Mortality differed considerably between PolyHeme and Control patients who had blunt injury and protocol violations (see **Table 4**). By comparison, the mortality between PolyHeme and Control patients sustaining penetrating wounds was virtually identical, whereas the distribution of major protocol violations was equivalent.

Exposure to allogeneic stored blood was a secondary efficacy end point. In the initial 12 hours post injury, 238 (68%) PolyHeme patients did not require RBCs compared with 183 (50%) Control patients ($P<.001$). By day 1, 201 (57%) PolyHeme patients and 174 (48%) Control patients did not require RBCs ($P<.001$). In addition, the time to first exposure to RBCs in those patients who received RBCs was markedly different. The median time to first unit of RBCs in the PolyHeme group was 7.6 hours (453.0 minutes) compared with 1.5 hours (88.5 minutes) in Control. In the Per Protocol cohort, the median time to first unit of RBCs in the PolyHeme group was 14.1 hours (848.0 minutes) compared with 1.5 hours (89.0 minutes) in Control.

Incidence of MOF was low in this study and not significantly different between groups: 26 of 350 (7.4%) in the PolyHeme group versus 20 of 364 (5.5%) in Control. Of the patients who developed MOF, a similar proportion from each group received at least six units of RBCs (PolyHeme 23/26, Control 18/20). There was a strong association in both groups between receiving six or more units of RBCs in the first 12 hours post trauma and MOF (PolyHeme odds ratio: 6.76; $P<.001$; Control odds ratio: 4.83, $P = .002$), as was found by the authors previously.[36]

Safety Analyses

As expected in seriously injured patients, AEs were reported in virtually all: 93% (324/349) of PolyHeme patients and 88% (322/365) of Control patients ($P = .041$). Investigator-reported AEs occurring in 20% or more of patients included anemia, pyrexia, hypocalcemia, hypokalemia, hyperglycemia, thrombocytopenia, leukocytosis, and tachycardia. SAEs were reported in 40% (141/349) of PolyHeme patients and in 35% (126/365) of Control patients ($P = .122$; **Table 5**).

Hypertension (**Table 6**) was reported more frequently as an AE in the PolyHeme group compared with Control (18% versus 12%, $P = .028$); however, the overall incidence of substantially abnormal episodes of systolic and diastolic hypertension on arrival to the hospital or through 6 hours post injury was low (5% PolyHeme versus 3% Control and 7% PolyHeme versus 7% Control, respectively). The lack of significant evidence of vasoconstriction is consistent with the authors' previous work.[27] The incidence of renal failure was also low and comparable between groups (3% in PolyHeme versus 2% in Control). There was also no difference in the incidence of nausea (17% in PolyHeme versus 15% in Control) or vomiting (13% in PolyHeme versus 12% in Control). Hyperamylasemia was reported in one PolyHeme patient versus no Control patients, and acute pancreatitis was reported in one PolyHeme patient and in two Control patients.

The risk of adverse myocardial-related events associated with HOBCs is particularly germane in light of a recent meta-analysis suggesting an increased risk of myocardial infarction (MI) with HBOCs in clinical trials.[71] There was no difference between groups in the incidence of combined cardiovascular events related to cardiac failure, malignant dysrhythmias, or cerebral ischemic/thrombotic complications (see **Table 5**).

Table 3
Baseline characteristics and demographics

Characteristic	As Randomized (N = 714)		As Treated (N = 714)		Per Protocol (N = 590)		Major Protocol Violations (N = 124)	
	PolyHeme (N = 350)	Control (N = 364)	PolyHeme (N = 349)	Control (N = 365)	PolyHeme (N = 279)	Control (N = 311)	PolyHeme (N = 71)	Control (N = 53)
Age (y)[a]	36.3 (0.8)	37.9 (0.9)	35.9 (0.8)	38.3 (0.9)	36.7 (0.9)	38.2 (0.9)	35.0 (1.7)	35.9 (2.3)
Age category (APACHE)[b]								
≤44 y	242 (69)	251 (69)	247 (71)	246 (67)	195 (70)	211 (68)	47 (66)	40 (76)
45–54 y	65 (19)	57 (16)	62 (18)	60 (16)	48 (17)	51 (16)	17 (24)	6 (11)
55–64 y	27 (8)	27 (7)	25 (7)	29 (8)	21 (8)	24 (8)	6 (9)	3 (6)
65–74 y	11 (3)	16 (4)	10 (3)	17 (5)	10 (4)	14 (5)	1 (1)	2 (4)
≥75 y	5 (1)	13 (4)	5 (1)	13 (4)	5 (2)	11 (4)	0 (0)	2 (4)
Male[b]	272 (78)	289 (79)	268 (77)	293 (80)	218 (78)	252 (81)	54 (76)	37 (70)
Ethnicity[b]								
Caucasian	160 (46)	170 (47)	156 (45)	174 (48)	127 (46)	151 (49)	33 (47)	19 (36)
African American	124 (35)	120 (33)	124 (36)	120 (33)	97 (35)	102 (33)	27 (38)	18 (34)
Hispanic	53 (15)	61 (17)	57 (16)	57 (16)	43 (15)	48 (15)	10 (14)	13 (25)
Asian	10 (3)	7 (2)	9 (3)	8 (2)	9 (3)	4 (1)	1 (1)	3 (6)
Other	3 (<1)	6 (2)	3 (<1)	6 (2)	3 (1)	6 (2)	0	0

Height (cm)[a]	174.5 (0.6)	173.4 (0.6)	174.3 (0.6)	173.6 (0.6)	174.8 (0.7)	173.9 (0.6)	173.4 (1.7)	170.1 (2.3)
Weight (kg)[a]	82.4 (1.1)	83.2 (1.2)	82.6 (1.1)	83.0 (1.2)	82.9 (1.3)	84.0 (1.2)	80.0 (2.5)	78.1 (3.6)
BMI (kg/m²)[a]	27.0 (0.4)	27.7 (0.4)	27.1 (0.3)	27.6 (0.4)	27.1 (0.4)	27.9 (0.4)	26.5 (0.9)	26.6 (1.2)
ISS[a]	19.9 (0.8)	19.4 (0.7)	20.1 (0.7)	19.2 (0.7)	19.1 (0.8)	19.1 (0.8)	22.9 (1.9)	21.2 (1.9)
ISS category[b]								
Mild/moderate (<9)	56 (16)	60 (16)	51 (15)	65 (18)	47 (17)	53 (17)	9 (13)	7 (13)
Serious (9–15)	107 (31)	101 (28)	107 (31)	101 (28)	87 (31)	90 (29)	20 (28)	11 (21)
Severe (16–24)	61 (17)	74 (20)	60 (17)	75 (21)	51 (18)	67 (22)	10 (14)	7 (14)
Critical/maximal (25–75)	126 (36)	123 (34)	129 (37)	120 (33)	94 (34)	99 (32)	32 (45)	24 (49)
Maximal (36–75)	48 (14)	41 (11)	46 (13)	43 (12)	36 (13)	36 (12)	12 (17)	5 (9)
Unsurvivable (75)	3 (<1)	1 (<1)	3 (<1)	1 (<1)	1 (<1)	1 (<1)	2 (3)	0
Mechanism of injury[b]								
Blunt	166 (47)	174 (48)	165 (47)	175 (48)	138 (49)	154 (50)	28 (39)	20 (40)
Penetrating	184 (53)	186 (52)	183 (53)	187 (52)	141 (51)	156 (50)	43 (61)	30 (60)
Transport mode[b]								
Air	121 (35)	122 (34)	117 (34)	126 (35)	99 (35)	112 (36)	22 (31)	10 (19)
Ground	229 (65)	242 (66)	232 (66)	239 (65)	180 (65)	199 (64)	49 (69)	43 (81)
Median Transport Time (min)[a]	26	26	26	26	27	26	24	26
SBP randomization (mm Hg)[a]	77.9 (0.7)	77.8 (0.6)	77.2 (0.6)	78.4 (0.7)	77.2 (0.7)	77.3 (0.6)	82.5 (3.3)	82.5 (2.7)
SBP <60 mm Hg[b]	17 (5)	19 (5)	16 (5)	20 (6)	12 (4)	19 (6)	4 (6)	1 (2)
Zero/no SBP obtained[b]	30 (9)	19 (5)	27 (8)	22 (6)	0	0	27 (39)	22 (41)
GCS randomization[a]	13.7 (0.1)	13.6 (0.1)	13.7 (0.1)	13.7 (0.1)	13.8 (0.1)	13.7 (0.1)	13.4 (0.3)	13.3 (0.4)

(continued on next page)

Table 3
(continued)

Characteristic	As Randomized (N = 714)		As Treated (N = 714)		Per Protocol (N = 590)		Major Protocol Violations (N = 124)	
	PolyHeme (N = 350)	Control (N = 364)	PolyHeme (N = 349)	Control (N = 365)	PolyHeme (N = 279)	Control (N = 311)	PolyHeme (N = 71)	Control (N = 53)
GCS randomization category[b]								
≤5	4 (1)	2 (<1)	4 (1)	2 (<1)	0	0	4 (6)	2 (4)
6–8	17 (5)	18 (5)	18 (5)	17 (5)	15 (5)	17 (5)	2 (3)	1 (2)
9–12	35 (10)	49 (13)	34 (10)	50 (14)	28 (10)	40 (13)	7 (10)	9 (17)
13–15	294 (84)	295 (81)	293 (84)	296 (81)	236 (85)	254 (82)	58 (82)	41 (77)
Hb at randomization (g/dL)[a,c]	13.2 (0.2)	13.0 (0.2)	13.2 (0.2)	13.0 (0.2)	13.3 (0.2)	13.0 (0.2)	12.8 (0.6)	12.7 (0.7)
PT at randomization (s)[a]	29.4 (2.6)[d]	20.9 (1.7)	29.8 (2.6)[d]	20.0 (1.6)	28.3 (2.8)[d]	20.2 (1.7)	37.4 (8.2)	28.5 (7.5)
aPTT at randomization (s)[a]	67.4 (7.3)[d]	46.6 (4.4)	68.6 (7.2)[d]	44.3 (4.2)	63.8 (7.7)[d]	43.1 (4.1)	92.6 (22.0)	80.1 (24.0)
Hb at ED admission (g/dL)[a,b]	12.3 (0.1)[d]	11.5 (0.2)	12.3 (0.1)[d]	11.5 (0.2)	12.5 (0.2)[d]	11.4 (0.2)	11.6 (0.4)	11.8 (0.4)
PT at ED admission (s)[a]	20.7 (1.2)	21.0 (1.3)	20.7 (1.2)	20.9 (1.3)	20.1 (1.3)	21.0 (1.4)	23.4 (3.1)	20.3 (2.7)
aPTT at ED admission (s)[a]	49.4 (3.8)	49.3 (4.1)	49.3 (3.7)	49.4 (4.1)	46.0 (3.9)	49.3 (4.5)	63.2 (10.1)	49.0 (9.2)

Research board approved the informed consent document and procedures. Additional protection of the rights and welfare of the subjects include community consultation, public disclosure, and establishment of an independent data monitoring committee. Consent to continue the study is obtained from the patient as soon as possible.

Abbreviations: aRTT, Activated partial thromboplastin time; ED, Emergency department; PT, Prothrombin time.

[a] Values are expressed as mean (SE).
[b] Values are expressed as n (%); percentages are based on the number of patients in each treatment group divided by number of patients who have nonmissing values.
[c] To convert to g/L, multiply by 0.1.
[d] P<0.05 compared with Control.

Data from Moore EE, Moore FA, Fabian TC, et al. Human polymerized hemoglobin for the treatment of hemorrhagic shock when blood is unavailable: the USA Multicenter Trial. J Am Coll Surg 2009;208:1–13.

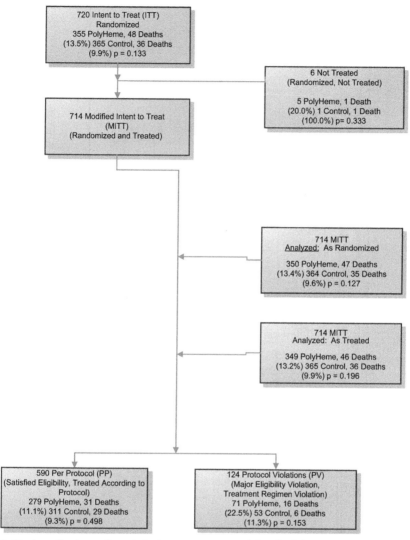

Fig. 8. Study patient enrollment. Patients were assessed for eligibility by paramedics in the field at the scene of injury; 722 patients were enrolled in the study. Two patients had their data withheld by the local institutional review board. The Modified Intent to Treat (MITT) population comprises 720 patients. The MITT population is analyzed two ways: "As Randomized," in which patients are analyzed in the group to which they were randomized (regardless of which treatment the patients received), and "As Treated," in which patients are analyzed according to the treatment they actually received. Of the 720 patients, 590 satisfied all the eligibility criteria and were treated according to the protocol; 124 violated eligibility criteria or did not adhere to the treatment regimen described in the protocol. (*Adapted from* Moore EE, Moore FA, Fabian TC, et al. Human polymerized hemoglobin for the treatment of hemorrhagic shock when blood is unavailable: the USA Multicenter Trial. J Am Coll Surg 2009;208:1–13; with permission.)

Table 4
Day 30 mortality by subgroups

Characteristic	As Randomized (N = 714)		As Treated (N = 14)		Per Protocol (N = 590)		Major Protocol Violations (N = 124)	
	PolyHeme (N = 350)	Control (N = 364)	PolyHeme (N = 349)	Control (N = 365)	PolyHeme (N = 279)	Control (N = 311)	PolyHeme (N = 71)	Control (N = 53)
Mortality by mechanism of injury[a]								
Blunt	30/166 (18.1)[d]	18/174 (10.3)	30/165 (18.2)[d]	18/175 (10.3)	22/138 (15.9)	17/154 (11.0)	8/28 (28.6)	1/20 (5.0)
Penetrating	17/184 (9.2)	17/186 (9.1)	16/183 (8.7)	18/187 (9.6)	9/141 (6.4)	12/156 (7.7)	8/43 (18.6)	5/30 (16.7)
Mortality by ISS category[a,b]								
Mild/moderate (1–8)	1/56 (1.8)	1/60 (1.7)	0/51 (0)	2/65 (3.1)	0/47 (0)	0/53 (0)	1/9 (11.1)	1/7 (14.3)
Serious (9–15)	4/107 (3.7)	2/101 (2.0)	4/107 (3.7)	2/101 (2.0)	3/87 (3.4)	2/90 (2.2)	1/20 (5.0)	0/11 (0)
Severe (16–24)	8/61 (13.1)	5/74 (6.8)	8/60 (13.3)	5/75 (6.7)	6/51 (11.8)	4/67 (6.0)	2/10 (20.0)	1/7 (14.3)
Critical (25–75)	34/126 (27.0)	25/123 (20.3)	33/129 (25.6)	26/120 (21.7)	22/94 (23.4)	22/99 (22.2)	12/32 (37.5)	3/24 (12.5)
Mortality regression model interaction terms[c]								
By randomization SBP	0.687		0.751		0.919		ND	
By APACHE age category	0.333		0.236		0.462		ND	
By mechanism of injury	0.187		0.146		0.350		ND	
By ISS	0.981		0.645		0.863		ND	
By GCS	0.536		0.703		0.172		ND	
By prerandomization crystalloid	0.194		0.106		0.101		ND	
By sex	0.312		0.914		0.779		ND	

Abbreviation: ND, Not determined.

[a] Values are expressed as number of deaths (%).

[b] Six patients did not have an ISS calculated: four were patients who had non-trauma-related blood loss; two were trauma patients who died early post injury and had inadequate documentation of their injuries.

[c] P values.

[d] P<.05 compared with Control.

Data from Moore EE, Moore FA, Fabian TC, et al. Human polymerized hemoglobin for the treatment of hemorrhagic shock when blood is unavailable: the USA Multicenter Trial. J Am Coll Surg 2009;208:1–13.

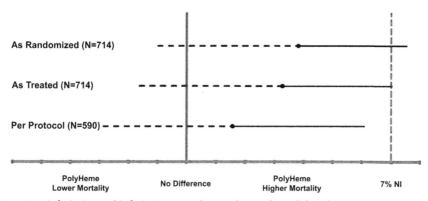

Fig. 9. Noninferiority and inferiority mortality analyses. The *solid circle* represents the point estimate for the observed mortality difference between the PolyHeme and Control groups for each cohort. The *dashed black line* represents the one-sided inferiority analysis using a final critical alpha level of 0.0144, having split the 0.05 starting alpha level using the Pocock spending function approach between four planned interim analyses and one final analysis. The *solid black line* represents the one-sided noninferiority (NI) analysis using a final critical alpha level of 0.044, having split the 0.05 starting alpha level using the O'Brien-Fleming spending function approach, as described by Lan and DeMets,[63] between one planned interim analysis for superiority after 500 patients had been enrolled and one final analysis. "7%NI" and the vertical *red dashed line* refer to the noninferiority boundary at 7% higher mortality in the PolyHeme group compared with Control. The As Randomized cohort includes the 714 patients (350 PolyHeme, 364 Control); the As Treated cohort includes 714 patients (349 PolyHeme, 365 Control); and the Per Protocol cohort includes 590 patients (279 PolyHeme, 311 Control). (*Adapted from* Moore EE, Moore FA, Fabian TC, et al. Human polymerized hemoglobin for the treatment of hemorrhagic shock when blood is unavailable: the USA Multicenter Trial. J Am Coll Surg 2009;208:1–13; with permission.)

The number of investigator-reported MIs was 11 in the PolyHeme group versus three in Control; none was considered by the investigator to be "possibly" or "probably" related to PolyHeme. Three MIs in the PolyHeme group did not fit the classic clinical profile: two were not substantiated by ECGs, enzymes, or autopsy reports and a third followed ligation of a coronary artery during repair of a ventricular stab wound. Cardiology recommended cardiac catheterization for one patient in each group; otherwise, no interventions were necessary. Three PolyHeme patients and one Control patient who had MIs died by day 30; the cause of death was MI in two patients (a 55-year-old man on day 1 and a 56-year-old man on day 19), cardiac arrhythmia in one patient (an 88-year-old woman on day 8), and MOF in one patient (a 63-year-old man on day 30). This overall low incidence of MI (2%) contrasts with the high rate of abnormal ECGs (75% in PolyHeme, 78% in Control), markedly abnormal creatine kinase–myocardial band (CK-MB) isoenzymes (65% in PolyHeme, 68% in Control), and markedly abnormal troponin I (26% in PolyHeme, 19% in Control).

Because of the disparity between high rates of ECG abnormalities and troponin and CK-MB elevation but low MI incidence, a post hoc independent Cardiac Event Subcommittee of experts in cardiology and resuscitation medicine blinded to treatment was convened to adjudicate these results. The committee developed a standardized decision algorithm to classify study patients as to the likelihood of MI (**Fig. 10**). Patients were stratified by chest trauma (defined as chest abbreviated injury score [AIS] ≤2 or >2). Patients who had an AIS of two or less were classified as having "absent infarction," "indeterminate infarction," "possible infarction," "probable

Table 5
Investigator-reported adverse events

Event	As Treated (N = 714)	
	PolyHeme (N = 349)	Control (N = 365)
AEs	324 (93)[b]	322 (88)
SAEs	141 (40)	126 (35)
Most common SAEs (>2%)		
Pneumonia	27 (8)	21 (6)
Hemorrhagic shock	20 (6)	16 (4)
Respiratory failure	21 (6)	17 (5)
Hypercoagulable state	18 (5)	12 (3)
Coagulopathy	13 (4)[b]	4 (1)
Sepsis	12 (3)	11 (3)
MI	10 (3)[b]	2 (1)
MI AEs[a]	11 (3)[b]	3 (1)
MI	7	2
NSTEMI	3	0
Non–Q wave MI	0	1
Acute traumatic MI	1	0
Requiring intervention	1	1
Death within 30 d	3	1
Cardiovascular events		
Heart failure/CHF/PE/fluid overload/ hypervolemia	20 (6)	20 (5)
Cardiac arrest/EMD/VFib/V-arrhythmia/VT	15 (4)	9 (2)
CVA/cerebral ischemia/cerebral infarction	3 (1)	1 (1)
MOF in 30 d (adjudicated)	26 (7)	20 (6)
Renal (creatinine >1.8 mg/dL)	13/26 (50)	9/20 (45)
Hepatic (total bilirubin >2.0 mg/dL)	20/26 (77)	15/20 (75)
Cardiac (inotropes)	9/26 (35)	4/20 (20)
Pulmonary (Pao_2/Fio_2 <240)	24/26 (92)	19/20(95)

Values are expressed as n (%): the number of patients who had the event divided by the total number of patients in each treatment group.

Abbreviations: CHF, Congestive heart failure; CVA, Cerebrovascular accident; EMD, Electromechanical dissociation; Fio_2, Fraction of inspired oxygen; MI, Myocardial infarction; NSTEMI, Non–ST-segment MI; PE, Pulmonary embolism; V, Ventricular; VFib, Ventricular fibrillation; VT, Ventricular tachycardia.

[a] Two MI events were not considered "serious" by the investigator.

[b] $P<.05$ compared with Control.

Data from Moore EE, Moore FA, Fabian TC, et al. Human polymerized hemoglobin for the treatment of hemorrhagic shock when blood is unavailable: the USA Multicenter Trial. J Am Coll Surg 2009;208:1–13.

infarction," or "physiologic stress or possible infarction." Patients who had an AIS greater than two were classified as having "absent infarction or injury," "indeterminate infarction or injury," "possible infarction or injury," "probable infarction or injury," or "physiologic stress or possible infarction or injury." The addition of the term "injury" to the possible and probable classifications of patients who had an AIS greater than two was done in recognition of the fact that chest trauma in and of itself can cause

Table 6
Systemic blood pressure

	As Treated (N = 714)		Per Protocol (N = 590)	
Characteristic	PolyHeme (N = 350)	Control (N = 364)	PolyHeme (N = 279)	Control (N = 311)
Markedly abnormal high SBP (>180 mm Hg)				
At admission[a]	6 (2)	5 (1)	5 (2)	4 (1)
At 6 h post injury[a]	11 (3)	5 (1)	10 (4)	4 (1)
At admission or 6 h post inury[a]	16 (5)	10 (3)	14 (5)	8 (3)
Markedly abnormal high DBP (>105 mm Hg)				
At admission[a]	23 (7)	18 (5)	17 (6)	14 (5)
At 6 h post injury[a]	3 (1)	8 (2)	3 (1)	5 (2)
At admission or 6 h post inury[a]	26 (7)	25 (7)	20 (7)	18 (6)
SBP at admission (mm Hg)[b]	115 (2)	113 (2)	115 (2)	113 (2)
SBP at 6 h post injury (mm Hg)[b]	129 (2)[c]	122 (2)	129 (2)[c]	122 (2)
DBP at admission (mm Hg)[b]	71 (1)[c]	68 (1)	71 (1)	68 (1)
DBP at 6 h post injury (mm Hg)[b]	73 (1)[c]	66 (1)	73 (1)[c]	66 (1)

Abbreviations: DPB, Diastolic blood pressure.
[a] Values are expressed as n (%); percentages are based on the number of patients in each treatment group divided by number of patients who had nonmissing values.
[b] Values are expressed as mean (SE).
[c] $P<.05$ compared with Control.
Data from Moore EE, Moore FA, Fabian TC, et al. Human polymerized hemoglobin for the treatment of hemorrhagic shock when blood is unavailable: the USA Multicenter Trial. J Am Coll Surg 2009;208:1–13.

elevations of cardiac enzymes and biomarkers in addition to abnormal ECGs.[72,73] Standardized methods of assessing ischemia/infarction on ECG recordings using ST elevation, ST depression, and T wave changes; ECG changes associated with prior MI; and left bundle branch block were employed. When a single abnormal ECG or biomarker was available before the patient died, the patient was classified as "possible infarction." When a patient had a cardiac arrest before an ECG or laboratory results were obtained, the patient was classified as indeterminate infarction, with a footnote that the patient died before testing. Each case was reviewed initially by two subcommittee members. In the event that classifications by these two members differed, all members reviewed the case. The final classification was determined by consensus.

The committee found a higher incidence of probable infarction in patients who had or did not have chest trauma than was reported by the investigators (**Table 7**). More patients were designated probable infarction in the PolyHeme group. The committee also reported the incidence of possible infarction in patients who did or did not have chest injury. When all of the categories of probable and possible infarction were grouped together, more than half of the patients in each group had some evidence of MI. The patients who had these combined designations were numerically higher in Control (193 [55.3%] patients versus 190 [52.1%] patients). There were more patients who had absent infarction in the PolyHeme group (84 versus 64) and more patients who had indeterminate infarction in Control (72 versus 111). In summary, a relationship of PolyHeme to elevated cardiac biomarkers and abnormal ECG findings was not supported by the data. A relationship of PolyHeme to MI could not be

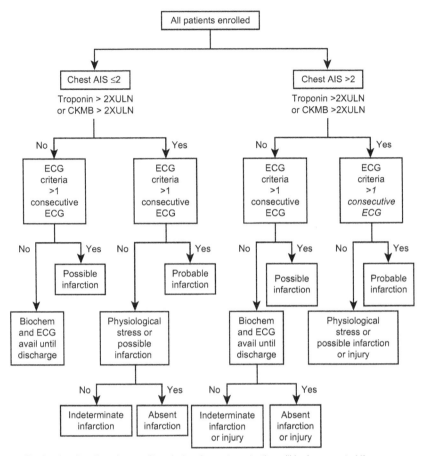

Regional wall motion abnormality or ischemia on stress testing will be incorporated if available.

Fig.10. MI algorithm. An independent data monitoring committee cardiac subcommittee reviewed all patient records in the Modified Intent to Treat–As Randomized cohort in a treatment-blinded fashion. Patients were assigned an MI category according to the algorithm based on ECG criteria and chest abbreviated injury score (AIS), troponin, and CK-MB data. 2XULN, two times upper limit of normal. (*Adapted from* Moore EE, Moore FA, Fabian TC, et al. Human polymerized hemoglobin for the treatment of hemorrhagic shock when blood is unavailable: the USA Multicenter Trial. J Am Coll Surg 2009;208:1–13; with permission.)

clearly ascertained from the totality of the cardiac data in this study, despite the higher number of investigator-reported MIs.

CLINICAL IMPLICATIONS OF THE PHASE III PREHOSPITAL HBOC RESUSCITATION TRIAL

Mortality at day 1 or day 30 was not statistically different between injured patients in shock who received up to six units of PolyHeme in lieu of blood for up to 12 hours following injury and Control patients who received the standard of care, including early blood transfusion. Mortality is best understood in the context of the novel study design and conduct of this trial, which presented multiple challenges. The protocol specified

Table 7
Independent Data Safety Monitoring Cardiac Sub committee Assignation of Myocardial infarction

| | As Treated (n = 714) | | | |
| | PolyHeme (n = 349) | | Control (n = 365) | |
Cardiac Committee Determination	n	%	n	%
Chest AIS ≤ 2				
Probable infarction	19	5.4	11	3.0
Physiologic stress or possible infarction	58	16.6	67	18.4
Possible infarction	5	1.4	6	1.6
Total possible or probable infarction	82	23.4	84	23.0
Absent infarction	61	17.5	52	14.2
Indetermine infarction	49	14.0	79	21.6
Chest AIS > 2				
Probable infarction or injury	23	6.6	19	5.2
Physiologic stress or possible infarction or injury	81	23.2	80	21.9
Possible infarction or injury	1	0.3	6	1.6
Total possible or probable infarction or injury	105	30.1	105	28.8
Absent infarction or injury	22	6.3	12	3.3
Indetermine infarction or injury	30	8.6	33	9.0

Values expressed as n (%); percentages are based on the number of patients in each treatment group divided by number of patients who had nonmissing values.
Data from Moore EE, Moore FA, Fabian TC, et al. Human polymerized hemoglobin for the treatment of hemorrhagic shock when blood is unavailable: the USA Multicenter Trial. J Am Coll Surg 2009;208:1–13.

enrollment of patients who were bleeding and in shock; therefore, it was necessary to conduct the study under federal regulation 21§CFR50.24, allowing an exception from informed consent.[60] In addition, the choice of the control group and the basis for statistical assessment of efficacy were complex. The ideal control group to assess efficacy of an oxygen carrier when blood is not available would comprise severely injured, massively bleeding patients who have critically low [Hb] levels and substantially delayed access to blood and the resulting high mortality. Prior clinical experience with PolyHeme in hospitalized patients[26–28,48,49,52,74–78] has shown that PolyHeme can provide life-sustaining oxygen-carrying capacity at otherwise life-threatening Hb levels.[52] Because of the possibility that the control group would include patients who had mixed injury severity, variable volumes of blood loss, and early access to blood, dual primary end points of superiority and noninferiority were employed. Thus, Control patients not sustaining critical anemia would not represent the scientifically appropriate control in which statistical superiority would be anticipated; such is the basis for extrapolating the observed results to the intended population.

Superiority in day 30 survival was not observed, likely due to several factors: short transport times, enrollment of patients who were not severely injured (only 34% of the Control group required more than six units of RBCs in the first 12 hours), and the occurrence of protocol violations. In the Per Protocol population, the results fell within the 7% noninferiority boundary, with a mortality difference of two patients between groups. The Per Protocol population represents the clearest opportunity to assess potential treatment effects because all other variables are well matched. The difference between the Per Protocol and As Randomized outcomes is influenced by patients who had major prespecified protocol violations (17%) related to eligibility or treatment regimen in this open-label study. **Tables 5** and **6** illustrate that more Poly-Heme patients had indicators of poor prognosis on enrollment, indicating potential futile resuscitation efforts. This is most evident in the subset of Major Protocol Violations patients who had blunt injury; a close review of this subset highlights an imbalance in critical variables between the PolyHeme and Control groups. The Major Protocol Violations patients receiving PolyHeme were characterized by higher ISS (31 versus 26), by lower randomization SBP (80 mm Hg versus 97 mm Hg), by lower randomization GCS (12 versus 14), and by more severe acidosis on arrival to the hospital (base deficit −8.8 mEq/L versus −6.5 mEq/L)—all of which correlate with a higher mortality. PolyHeme administration cannot influence ISS, randomization SBP, or GCS because these are obtained before infusion. Furthermore, more Poly-Heme patients than Control patients had markedly abnormal coagulation status (prothrombin time >17seconds) on enrollment (29% versus 20%). This clinical observation is important and is another potential indication of difference in injury severity. The imbalances in these critical variables alone could potentially account for the observed mortality difference between PolyHeme and Control in the blunt-injury Major Protocol Violations patients.

Transfusion avoidance is particularly relevant to the intended use of PolyHeme for treatment until definitive care and blood become available. Transfusion of six units of allogeneic blood in the first 12 hours has been invoked as the dominant risk factor in the development of postinjury MOF.[32,36] PolyHeme has been shown to attenuate the immunoinflammatory effects of stored RBCs,[47-49] forming the basis for infusing up to six units of PolyHeme in 12 hours. PolyHeme patients had a statistically significant reduction in the incidence of blood use during the 12- and 24-hour intervals. Although there was no difference in MOF between the groups, 23 of 26 PolyHeme patients and 18 of 20 Control patients who developed MOF also received six units of banked blood. Conceivably, higher allowed doses of PolyHeme within the 12-hour therapeutic window, in lieu of blood, might have reduced the incidence of MOF by averting the adverse immunoinflammatory effects of stored RBCs.

Safety of HBOCs remains a topic of considerable debate.[71] The early history with HBOCs included efforts to remove the stromal contaminants believed to be responsible for the observed safety concerns. Savitsky and colleagues,[79] however, described vasoconstriction and organ dysfunction in healthy volunteers with a stroma-free tetrameric Hb preparation. Subsequent efforts have focused on removal of small molecular weight tetrameric Hb as a way of improving safety.[2,7] In addition, there has been considerable attention paid to the adverse experiences with HBOCs and the potential mechanisms of NO scavenging,[9-11,80-81] the generation of reactive oxygen species,[3] and reflex autoregulation.[6] PolyHeme is polymerized to improve intravascular persistence and then purified to remove virtually all unpolymerized tetramer (<1%) and decrease the interactions with NO that could lead to vasoconstriction.[82-90]

Safety data in **Table 7** show a higher incidence of AEs and SAEs in the PolyHeme group. Of particular concern was that investigators reported more MIs in the Poly-Heme group in this open-label study, although the overall low incidence of MI contrasts with the high incidence of enzymes, biomarkers, and abnormal ECGs. Because of the disparity between high numbers of reported ECG abnormalities and troponin and CK-MB elevation but low reported MI rates, an independent Cardiac Event Subcommittee was convened to adjudicate these results. The committee found a higher incidence of probable infarction in patients who had or did not have chest trauma than was reported by the investigators. More patients were designated probable infarction in the PolyHeme group. The committee also reported the incidence of possible infarction in patients who had and did not have chest injury. When all of the categories of probable and possible infarction were grouped together, more than half of the patients in each group had some evidence of MI. Troponin elevations have been reported in 29% to 44% of critically ill and trauma populations.[72,73] Because blood samples and ECGs were obtained serially in this study following admission, the high rates of CK-MB, troponin, and abnormal ECGs may reflect the transitory sequelae of chest trauma in many of these patients rather than myocardial ischemia due to coronary artery disease. Furthermore, analysis of a comprehensive grouping of cardiovascular AEs shows no difference between the groups in the incidence of events related to ischemia, pump failure, or dysrhythmias. Incidences of significant hypertensive episodes and renal failure were low and comparable between groups.

Safety must be assessed in the context of the potential benefit of PolyHeme; that is, improved survival in patients who have life-threatening Hb levels when blood is not available or not an option. This benefit was demonstrated in prior clinical experience with PolyHeme in hospitalized patients[26–28,48,49,52,74] and in multiple emergency, compassionate treatments.[75,77,78] The results from this study suggest some increase in frequency of AEs compared with the use of blood. Consequently, PolyHeme would not be used interchangeably with RBCs but would be used when the likelihood of dying without oxygen-carrying replacement is so great that the potential life-sustaining benefit would exceed any potential risks. A recent meta-analysis pooled data from multiple different products used in multiple different clinical settings and concluded that there was no role for any of the HBOCs currently in clinical development.[71] Such a statistical tool of meta-analysis comparing various products under the umbrella of an entire class can be a useful tool to raise questions that merit answers with respect to the class; however, meta-analysis is not designed to provide answers about specific products or to examine fully the risk-to-benefit ratio of any particular product, particularly for the intended clinical use.[91] Rather, that is the role of clinical trials such as the current study with PolyHeme that are focused and con-ducted to assess the safety and efficacy in relation to a proposed indication—in this case, an indication that addresses a critical, unmet need when there is no available alternative. In this setting, it is possible for an HBOC such as PolyHeme to provide a clinically meaningful benefit, even though the outcome may be less favorable than would be seen with stored blood.

There is an undisputed need for a universally compatible, oxygen-carrying product with long-term storage capability and reduced risk of disease transmission for use when RBCs are not available or not an option. Military battlefield casualties,[92] disaster scenarios,[93] blood incompatibility and shortages, and religious objection[94] represent additional situations in which PolyHeme can address this critical unmet medical need. The combination of PolyHeme's life-sustaining capability, the logistic benefits, and the acceptable benefit-to-risk calculus for the intended indication represents an opportu-nity to provide an alternative to transfusion for patients at high risk of death when stored RBCs are not available.

REFERENCES

1. Department of Health and Human Services/US Food and Drug Administration. Biologics Licensing 21 CFR601.25(d) (2). Federal Register April 1, 2004.
2. Points to consider in the safety evaluation of hemoglobin-based oxygen carriers. Center for Biologics Evaluation and Research. Transfusion 1991;31:369–71.

3. Alayash AI. Oxygen therapeutics—can we tame hemoglobin? Nat Rev Drug Discov 2004;3:152–9.
4. Creteur J, Sibbald W, Vincent JL. Hemoglobin solutions—not just red blood cell substitutes. Crit Care Med 2000;28:3025–34.
5. McFaul SJ, Bowman PD, Villa VM. Hemoglobin stimulates the release of proinflammatory cytokines from leukocytes in whole blood. J Lab Clin Med 2000; 135:263–9.
6. Winslow RM. Current status of blood substitute research—towards a new paradigm. J Intern Med 2003;253:508–17.
7. Points to consider on efficacy evaluation of hemoglobin and perfluorocarbon based oxygen carriers. Center for Biologics Evaluation and Research. Transfusion 1994;34:712–3.
8. Sloan EP, Koenigsberg M, Gens D, et al. Diaspirin cross-linked hemoglobin (DCLHb) in the treatment of severe traumatic hemorrhagic shock—a randomized controlled efficacy trial. JAMA 1999;282:1857–64.
9. Hess JR, MacDonald VW, Brinkley WW. Systemic and pulmonary hypertension after resuscitation with cell-free hemoglobin. J Appl Phys 1993;74:1769–78.
10. Poli de Figueiredo LF, Mathru M, Solanki D, et al. Pulmonary hypertension and systemic vasoconstriction may offset the benefits of acellular hemoglobin blood substitutes. J Trauma 1997;42:847–56.
11. Gulati A, Sen AP, Sharma AC, et al. Role of ET and NO in resuscitative effect of diaspirin cross-linked hemoglobin after hemorrhage in rat. Am J Phys 1997; 273:H827–36.
12. Rohlfs RJ, Bruner E, Chiu A, et al. Arterial blood pressure responses to cell-free hemoglobin solutions and the reaction with nitric oxide. J Biol Chem 1998;273: 12128–34.
13. Schultz SC, Grady B, Cole F, et al. A role for endothelin and nitric oxide in the pressor response to diaspirin cross-linked hemoglobin. J Lab Clin Med 1993; 122:301–8.
14. Boura C, Caron A, Longrois D, et al. Volume expansion with modified hemoglobin solution, colloids, or crystalloid after hemorrhagic shock in rabbits: effects in skeletal muscle oxygen pressure versus arterial blood velocity and resistance. Shock 2003;19:176–82.
15. Wettstein R, Cabrales P, Erni D, et al. Resuscitation from hemorrhagic shock with MalPEG-albumin: comparison with MalPEG-hemoglobin. Shock 2004;22:351–7.
16. Fushitan K, Imai K, Riggs AF. Oxygen properties of hemoglobin from the earthworm Lumbricus terrestris. J Biol Chem 1986;261:8414–23.
17. Hirsch RE, Jelicks LA, Wittenberg BA, et al. A first evaluation of the natural high molecular weight polymeric Lumbricus terrestris hemoglobin as an oxygen carrier. Artif Cells Blood Substit Immobil Biotechnol 1997;25:429–44.
18. Levy JH, Goodnough LT, Greilich PE, et al. Polymerized bovine hemoglobin solution as a replacement for allogeneic red blood cell transfusion after cardiac surgery: results of a randomized, double-blind trial. J Thorac Cardiovasc Surg 2002;124:35–42.
19. LaMuraglia GM, O'Hara PJ, Baker WH, et al. The reduction of the allogenic transfusion requirement in aortic surgery with hemoglobin-based solution. J Vasc Surg 2000;31:299–308.
20. Standl T, Burmeister MA, Horn EP, et al. Bovine haemoglobin-based oxygen carrier for patients undergoing haemodilution before liver resection. Br J Anaesth 1998;80:189–94.

21. Kasper SM, Walter M, Grune F, et al. Effects of a hemoglobin-based oxygen carrier (HBOC-201) on hemodynamics and oxygen transport in patients undergoing preoperative hemodilution for elective abdominal aortic surgery. Anesth Analg 1996;83:921–7.
22. Hughes GS Jr, Antal EJ, Locker PK, et al. Physiology and pharmacokinetics of a novel hemoglobin-based oxygen carrier in humans. Crit Care Med 1996;24: 756–64.
23. Handrigan MT, Bentley TB, Oliver JD, et al. Choice of fluid influences outcome in prolonged hypotensive resuscitation after hemorrhage in awake rats. Shock 2005;23:337–43.
24. Manning JE, Katz LM, Brownstein MR, et al. Bovine hemoglobin-based oxygen carrier (HBOC-201) for resuscitation of uncontrolled, exsanguinating liver injury in swine. Shock 2000;13:152–9.
25. McNeil JD, Smith DL, Jenkins DH, et al. Hypotensive resuscitation using a polymerized bovine-based oxygen carrying solution leads to reversal of anaerobic metabolism. J Trauma 2001;50:1063–75.
26. Gould SA, Moore EE, Moore FA, et al. Clinical utility of human polymerized hemoglobin as a blood substitute after acute trauma and urgent surgery. J Trauma 1997;43:325–32.
27. Johnson JL, Moore EE, Offner PJ, et al. Resuscitation of the injured patient with polymerized stroma-free hemoglobin does not produce systemic or pulmonary hypertension. Am J Surg 1998;176:612–7.
28. Gould SA, Moore EE, Hoyt DB, et al. The first randomized trial of human polymerized hemoglobin as a blood substitute in acute trauma and emergent surgery. J Am Coll Surg 1998;187:113–22.
29. Botha AJ, Moore FA, Moore EE, et al. Postinjury neutrophil priming and activation—an early vulnerable window. Surgery 1995;118:358–65.
30. Ciesla DJ, Moore EE, Johnson JL, et al. A 12 year prospective study of postinjury multiple organ failure. Arch Surg 2005;140:432–40.
31. Aiboshi J, Moore EE, Ciesla DJ, et al. Blood transfusion and the two-insult model of postinjury multiple organ failure. Shock 2001;15:302–6.
32. Silliman CC, Moore EE, Johnson JL, et al. Transfusion of the injured patient: proceed with caution. Shock 2004;21:291–9.
33. Moore EE, Moore FA, Harken HA, et al. The two-event construct of postinjury multiple organ failure. Shock 2005;24:S71–4.
34. Ingraham LM, Allen JM, Higgins CP, et al. Metabolic membrane and functional responses of human polymorphonuclear leukocytes to platelet activating factor. Blood 1982;59:1259–66.
35. Souaia A, Moore FA, Moore EE, et al. Early predictors of post-injury multiple organ failure. Arch Surg 1994;129:38–45.
36. Moore FA, Moore EE, Sauaia A. Blood transfusion—an independent risk factor for postinjury multiple organ failure. Arch Surg 1997;132:620–5.
37. Zallen G, Offner PJ, Moore EE, et al. Age of transfused blood is an independent risk factor for post-injury multiple organ failure. Am J Surg 1999;178: 570–2.
38. Biffl WL, Moore EE, Zallen G, et al. Neutrophils are primed for cytotoxicity and resist apoptosis in injured patients at risk for multiple organ failure. Surgery 1999;126:198–202.
39. Bordin JO, Heddle NM, Blajchman MA. Biologic effects of leukocytes present in transfused cellular blood products. Blood 1994;84:1703–21.

40. Nielsen HJ, Reimert CM, Pedersen AM, et al. Time-dependent spontaneous release of white cell and platelet derived bioactive substances from stored human blood. Transfusion 1996;36:960–5.
41. Shanwell A, Dristiansson M, Remberger M, et al. Generation of cytokines in red cell concentrates during storage is prevented by pre-storage white cell reduction. Transfusion 1997;36:678–84.
42. Silliman CC, Paterson AJ, Dickey WO, et al. The association of biologically active lipids with the development of transfusion-related acute lung injury. Transfusion 1997;37:719–26.
43. Silliman CC, Voelkel NF, Allard JD, et al. Plasma and lipids from stored packed red blood cells cause acute lung injury in an animal model. J Clin Invest 1998; 101:1458–67.
44. Biffl WL, Moore EE, Offner PJ, et al. Plasma from aged stored red blood cells delays neutrophil apoptosis and primes for cytotoxicity: abrogation by post storage washing but not prestorage leukoreduction. J Trauma 2001;50:426–31 [discussion: 432].
45. Moore EE. Blood substitutes: the future is now. J Am Coll Surg 2003;196:1–17.
46. Partrick DA, Moore EE, Barnett CC, et al. Human polymerized hemoglobin as a blood substitute avoids transfusion-induced PMN priming for superoxide and elastase release. Shock 1997;7:24.
47. Masuno T, Moore EE, Cheng AM, et al. Prehospital hemoglobin based oxygen carrier (HBOC) resuscitation attenuates postinjury acute lung injury. Surgery 2005;B8:335–41.
48. Johnson JL, Moore EE, Offner PJ, et al. Resuscitation with a blood substitute abrogates pathologic postinjury neutrophil cytotoxic function. J Trauma 2004; 50:449–56.
49. Johnson JL, Moore EE, Gonzalez RJ, et al. Alteration of the postinjury hyperinflammatory response by means of resuscitation with a red cell substitute. J Trauma 2003;54:133–40.
50. Huston P, Peterson R. Withholding proven treatment in clinical research. N Engl J Med 2001;345:912–3.
51. McRae AD, Weijer C. Lessons from everyday lives: a moral justification for acute care research. Crit Care Med 2002;30:1146–51.
52. Gould SA, Moore EE, Hoyt DB, et al. The life-sustaining capacity of human polymerized hemoglobin when red cells may be available. J Am Coll Surg 2002;195:445–55.
53. Gawande A. Casualties of war—military care for the wounded from Iraq and Afghanistan. N Engl J Med 2004;351:2471–8.
54. Bickell WH, Wall MJ, Pepe PE, et al. Immediate versus delayed fluid resuscitation for hypotensive patients with penetrating torso injuries. N Engl J Med 1994;331: 1105–9.
55. Sondeen JL, Coopes VG, Holcomb JB. Blood pressure at which rebleeding occurs after resuscitation in swine and aortic injury. J Trauma 2004;54:S110–7.
56. Claridge JA, Schulman AM, Young JS. Improved resuscitation minimizes respiratory dysfunction and blunts interleukin-6 and nuclear factor-kB activation after traumatic shock. Crit Care Med 2002;30:1815–9.
57. Dunham CM, Siegel JH, Weitreter L, et al. Oxygen debt and metabolic acidemia as quantitative predictors of mortality and severity of the ischemic insult in hemorrhagic shock. Crit Care Med 1991;19:231–41.
58. Shoemaker WC, Appel PL, Kram HB. Tissue oxygen debt as a determinant of lethal and nonlethal postoperative organ failure. Crit Care Med 1988;16: 1117–20.

59. Moore EE, Moore FA, Fabian TC, et al. Human polymerized hemoglobin for the treatment of hemorrhagic shock when blood is unavailable: the USA Multicenter Trial. J Am Coll Surg 2009;208:1–13

60. Department of Health and Human Services/US Food and Drug Administration. Protection of human rights: informed consent and waiver of informed consent in certain emergency research. Final rules. 21 CFR Parts 50, 56, 312, 314, 601, 612, and 814. Federal Register 1996;61:51497–531.

61. Moore FA, McKinley BA, Moore EE, et al. Inflammation and the host response to injury, a large-scale collaborative project: guidelines for shock resuscitation. J Trauma 2006;61:82–9.

62. Dunnett CW, Gent M. Alternative to the use of two-sided tests in clinical trials. Stat Med 1996;15:1729–38.

63. Lan KKG, DeMets DL. Discrete sequential boundaries for clinical trials. Biometrika 1983;70:659–63.

64. Morikawa T, Yoshida M. A useful testing strategy in phase III trials: combined test of superiority and test of equivalence. J Biopharm Stat 1995;5:297–306.

65. O'Brien PC, Fleming TR. A multiple testing procedure for clinical trials. Biometrics 1979;35:549–56.

66. Pocock SJ. Group sequential methods in the design and analysis of clinical trials. Biometrika 1977;645:191–9.

67. Wang SK, Tsiatis AA. Approximately optimal one-parameter boundaries for group sequential trials. Biometrics 1987;43:193–9.

68. Heckbert SR, Vedder NB, Hoffman W, et al. Outcome after hemorrhagic shock in trauma patients. J Trauma 1998;45:545–9.

69. Mattox KL, Maningas PA, Moore EE, et al. Prehospital hypertonic saline/dextran infusion for post-traumatic hypotension. The USA Multicenter Trial. Ann Surg 1991;213:482–91.

70. Barkana Y, Stein M, Maor R, et al. Prehospital blood transfusion in prolonged evacuation. J Trauma 1999;45:176–80.

71. Natanson C, Kern SJ, Lurie P, et al. Cell-free hemoglobin-based blood substitutes and risk of myocardial infarction and death: a meta-analysis. JAMA 2008;299:2304–12.

72. Martin M, Mullenix P, Rhee P, et al. Troponin increases in the critically injured patients: mechanical trauma or physiologic stress? J Trauma 2005;58:1086–91.

73. Velmahos GC, Karaiskskis M, Salim A, et al. Normal electrocardiography and serum troponin I levels preclude the presence of clinically significant blunt cardiac injury. J Trauma 2004;54:45–51.

74. Moore EE, Cheng AM, Moore HB, et al. Hemoglobin-based oxygen carriers in trauma care: scientific rationale for the US Multicenter Prehospital Trial. World J Surg 2006;30:1247–57.

75. Cothern C, Moore EE, Offner PJ, et al. Bood substitute and erythropoietin therapy in severely anemic Jehovah's Witness. N Engl J Med 2002;346:1097–8.

76. Norris EJ, Ness PM, Williams GM. Use of a human polymerized hemoglobin solution as an adjunct to acute normovolemic hemodilution during complex abdominal aortic reconstruction. J Clin Anesth 2003;15:220–3.

77. Raff JP, Dobson CE, Tsai HM. Transfusion of polymerised human haemoglobin in a patient with severe sickle-cell anemia. Lancet 2002;360:454–65.

78. Smith SE, Toor A, Rodriquez T, et al. The administration of polymerized human hemoglobin (pyridoxylated) to a Jehovah's Witness after submyeloablative stem cell transplantation complicated by delayed graft failure. Compr Ther 2006;32:172–5.

79. Savitsky JP, Docze J, Black J, et al. A clinical trial of stroma-free hemoglobin. Clin Pharmacol Ther 1978;23:73–80.
80. Stamler JS, Jia L, Eu JP, et al. Blood flow regulation by S-nitrosohemoglobin in the physiological oxygen gradient. Science 1997;276:2034–7.
81. Yu B, Raher MJ, Volpato GP, et al. Inhaled nitric oxide enables artificial blood transfusion without hypertension. Circulation 2008;117:1982–90.
82. Gould SA, Moss GS. Clinical development of human polymerized hemoglobin as a blood substitute. World J Surg 1996;20:1200–7.
83. Gould SA, Rosen A, Sehgal L, et al. The effect of altered hemoglobin-oxygen affinity on oxygen transport by hemoglobin solution. J Surg Res 1980;28:246–51.
84. Gould SA, Rosen AL, Sehgal LR, et al. Polymerized pyridoxylated hemoglobin: efficacy as an O_2 carrier. J Trauma 1986;26:903–8.
85. Moss GS, Gould SA, Sehgal LR, et al. Hemoglobin solution—from tetramer to polymer. Surgery 1984;95:249–55.
86. Gould SA, Sehgal LR, Rosen AL, et al. The efficacy of polymerized pyridoxylated hemoglobin solution as an O_2 carrier. Ann Surg 1990;211:394–8.
87. Rosen AL, Gould SA, Sehgal LR, et al. Effect of hemoglobin solution on compensation to anemia in the erythrocyte-free primate. J Appl Phys 1990;68:938–43.
88. Sehgal LR, Rosen AL, Gould SA, et al. Preparation and in vitro characteristics of polymerized pyridoxylated hemoglobin. Transfusion 1983;23:158–62.
89. Sehgal LR, Gould SA, Rosen AL, et al. Polymerized pyridoxylated hemoglobin: a red cell substitute with normal oxygen capacity. Surgery 1984;95:433–8.
90. Wilkerson DK, Rosen AL, Sehgal LR, et al. Limits of cardiac compensation in anemic baboons. Surgery 1988;103:665–70.
91. LeLorier J, Gregoire G, Benhaddad A, et al. Discrepancies between meta-analyses and subsequent large randomized, controlled trials. N Engl J Med 1997;337:536–42.
92. Holcomb JB, McMullin NR, Pearse L, et al. Causes of death in the U.S. Special Operations Forces in the global war on terrorism. Ann Surg 2007;245:1–6.
93. Schimdt PJ. Blood and disaster: supply and demand. N Engl J Med 2002;346:617–20.
94. Carson JL, Noveck H, Berlin JA, et al. Mortality and morbidity in patients with very low postoperative Hb levels who decline blood transfusion. Transfusion 2002;42:812–8.

Design of Recombinant Hemoglobins for Use in Transfusion Fluids

Clara Fronticelli, PhD*, Raymond C. Koehler, PhD

KEYWORDS

- Blood substitute • Hemoglobin • Myoglobin
- Nitric oxide • Oxygen carrier • Transfusion

The need for transfusion fluids to treat a variety of clinical conditions is continually increasing. The use of acellular hemoglobin (Hb) solutions as a red blood cell (RBC) replacement is being evaluated.[1–5] Evolution maximizes the best conformational and functional characteristics of proteins as related to their natural in vivo function, and the role of the Hb molecule is best expressed when contained within the erythrocytes. The transformation of such a protein into an acellular oxygen carrier necessitates the introduction of functional and conformational modifications to optimize the characteristics of the protein to the different environmental conditions. In physiologic conditions, the oxygen affinity of the erythrocytes (P_{50} = 28 Torr) is lower than that of acellular Hb (P_{50} = 18 Torr). Solutions of stroma-free Hb contain tetrameric (molecular weight [MW] 64 kDa) and dimeric (MW 32 kDa) molecules at equilibrium. Due to the rapid filtration of the low-molecular-weight dimers through the kidneys, the retention time of infused acellular Hb is short.[6] In addition, Hb molecules can filter through the endothelium and scavenge nitric oxide (NO) from the interstitial fluid, producing the vasoconstriction observed upon administration of acellular Hb solutions.[7,8] Moreover, acellular Hb in the plasma facilitates the delivery of bound oxygen.[9,10] Under normal conditions, the increased perivascular PO_2 is thought to contribute to vasoconstriction and the associated increase in arterial pressure.[11,12] This vasoconstriction may prevent excessive oxygen delivery to the tissues and free radical formation. However, persistent constriction of upstream arterioles under conditions of hemorrhagic shock or partial ischemia due to facilitated precapillary oxygen loss by an Hb-based oxygen carrier (HBOC) can exert a counterproductive effect of RBC perfusion of the downstream capillary network.[13,14]

The authors were supported by a grant from the National Institute of Neurological Disorders and Stroke (NS-38684) and by the Eugene and Mary B. Meyer Center for Advanced Transfusion Practice and Blood Research at the Johns Hopkins University School of Medicine.

Department of Anesthesiology and Critical Care Medicine, The Johns Hopkins University School of Medicine, 600 North Wolfe Street, Blalock 1404, Baltimore, MD 21287, USA

* Corresponding author.

E-mail address: cfrontic@jhmi.edu (C. Fronticelli).

The following characteristics are necessary for an effective HBOC: (1) absence of renal filtration, (2) absence of NO scavenging effects, (3) stability toward auto-oxidation and heme loss, and (4) calibrated oxygen delivery. Clearly the development of an effective HBOC is a monumental task that will require contributions from basic science, animal experimentation, and clinical applications.

Chemical modifications are used to transform human and bovine Hbs into blood substitutes and large scale productions have been implemented. The first HBOCs, designed to have an oxygen affinity similar to blood and not to dissociate into dimers, were generated by introducing cross-links in the central cavity as the α-α fumaryl (HemAssist; Baxter Healthcare Corp., Deerfield, Illinois)[15] or by introducing pyridoxal phosphate to decrease the oxygen affinity combined with polymerization using glutaraldehyde to increase the molecular size (Polyheme; Northfield Laboratories Inc., Evanston, Illinois; Hemopure; Biopure Corp., Cambridge, Massachusetts).[16–19] More recent products are the zero-link bovine Hb (ZL-HbBv), which has large polymers formed in the absence of residual chemicals (Oxyvita, New Windsor, New York),[20] and Hb conjugated with polyethylene glycol (PEG) (Hemospan, Sangart; Sanguinate, Prolong Pharmaceuticals).[21–23] These more recent products have a high oxygen affinity, which may act to minimize vasoconstriction of the arterioles as a regulatory mechanism for excess oxygen delivery. In addition, solutions of pegylated Hb incorporate the characteristics of a plasma volume expander due to their high viscosity and oncotic pressure. The efficacy and potential adverse effects of these products for therapeutic applications are under rigorous scrutiny.[24]

RECOMBINANT HEMOGLOBIN

As an alternative approach to chemically modifying naturally occurring Hb, recombinant technology can be applied to the development of unique HBOCs. Hb can be expressed in microorganisms, and this approach eliminates the use of proteins of mammals, which may be in limited supply or may be infected by viruses or other pathogens. This technology offers the possibility for construction of mutant molecules that incorporate specific conformational and functional characteristics in the absence of chemical modifications.

Hemoglobin is a tetrameric protein composed of two structurally similar subunits, α and β, assembled through two different interfaces, $\alpha_1 \beta_1$ and $\alpha_1 \beta_2$. Each subunit contains eight α-helices (A–H) that form a pocket containing the heme. Tetrameric Hb is present in two states at equilibrium, deoxygenated (T) and oxygenated (R). Correct assembly of this protein requires expression of native α- and β-globins and their assembly and folding into the final quaternary structure upon combination with the heme. The first expression systems were developed by Kiyoshi Nagai and Hans Christian Thogersen[25] and adapted by Clara Fronticelli and colleagues.[26] In these systems, β-globin was expressed as a fusion protein with blood coagulation factor Xa. Cleavage of the isolated fusion protein released the authentic β-globin, which assembled into tetrameric Hb in the presence of native α-subunits and the heme. In a similar way, recombinant α-globin was expressed and assembled using native β-subunits.[27,28] Expression of soluble Hb was subsequently achieved by coexpressing the soluble α and β-chains in *Escherichia coli*, and several expression systems and purification procedures have been described.[29–31] The recombinant Hbs (rHbs) have functional characteristics similar to the natural protein and thus are apt to be molded for therapeutic applications as HBOCs.

A problem encountered in the development of rHbs as HBOCs is their low expression yield. Production of rHb in an amount sufficient for animal testing in an academic setting becomes too expensive, confining the in vivo experimentation to small animals and thus limiting the investigations and applications. The refolding of tetrameric Hb involves various steps: expression of α- and β-globins and their correct assembly into αβ dimers, reconstitution with heme, and final assembly into the functional tetrameric structure. An approach to improve the process is to increase the intrinsic stability of the expressed globins by using amino acid substitutions; however, this approach may modify the refolding pathway and not increase the yield of the protein.[32] An α-Hb stabilizing protein (AHSP) that has a protective effect toward the α-subunits has been identified.[33–35] William Brinigar at Temple University has incorporated a synthetic gene into a plasmid expressing only the α-globin and has observed the synthesis of α-globin (C. Fronticelli, personal communication, 2006). Conversely, α-globin was not expressed from an analogous plasmid that did not contain the AHSP gene. When AHSP was incorporated in the plasmid expressing α- and β-globins, however, an increase in the yield of rHb was not observed. Further investigation is necessary to understand the role of this chaperone in the control and stabilization of rHb. In their laboratory, the authors improved the expression yield of rHb by constructing a hybrid rHb, Hb Minotaur, using human α-globin and bovine β-globin.[36] The authors observed that bovine β-globin was considerably more resistant to denaturation than the human β-globin. With this plasmid, bovine β-globin was expressed significantly more than human α-globin. To help balance the production of α-globin with β-globin, a second α-globin gene was inserted in the plasmid and the amount of Hb isolated was much increased.

A major problem encountered on transfusion of acellular tetrameric Hb is its dissociation into dimers and the associated nephrotoxicity. The first step in the construction of an HBOC from rHb for therapeutic applications consisted of the construction of an expression vector that contained one gene encoding the β-globin and one gene that contained two copies of the α-globin, fused together by a single codon encoding glycine residues.[29] The low oxygen affinity (P_{50} = 32 Torr) of this Hb, referred to as rHb1.1, was attained by substituting asparagine for lysine at the β108 position on human Hb. The fused α-chains prevented dimer formation and renal filtration. Transfusion into beagle dogs resulted in a fourfold increase in the plasma retention time and maintenance of renal function, thereby demonstrating the validity of this approach in solving the nephrotoxicity problem. However, the stabilized tetramers were still small enough to extravasate in vascular beds without tight endothelial junctions.

HEME-POCKET MUTATIONS

To transform an Hb molecule into an HBOC, it is necessary to introduce into the molecule elements of ligand control and discrimination, high affinity for the heme, and resistance to auto-oxidation. John Olson[37,38] and collaborators at Rice University, taking as a model compound the monomeric myoglobin (Mb) molecule, have addressed these essential issues by investigating the effect of various heme-pocket mutations. Oxygen affinity can be decreased up to 100 fold by alteration of the H-bond between N^ϵ-His E7 and bound oxygen, with replacement of His E7 with Gly, Ala, Val, Ile, Leu, or Phe. Auto-oxidation was decreased, with stabilization of bound oxygen, with the mutation Leu(29) → Phe that introduces favorable electrostatic interaction with bound oxygen. Heme affinity was increased by strengthening the polar interaction with residues in the heme pocket.

The final steps of Mb refolding in vivo require precise interrelationships between the rates of protein synthesis, folding, and heme binding. If this synchronism is altered, the heme pocket does not attain its final structure.[39] Therefore, the overall complexity of this approach is evident and is compounded when applied to tetrameric Hb that has two nonidentical α and β pockets, in which the correlation of conformational and functional events governs the allosteric properties of the protein.

As an example of this complexity, the authors reported data from their laboratory on the different effects of modified heme-pocket polarity in Hb. Access of ligands to the heme group is hindered by the presence of the globin chain, which buries the heme in a hydrophobic crevice. The Hb heme pocket is lined by hydrophobic residues, except for the proximal (F8) and distal (E7) histidines, which are critical to the functional properties. The authors modified the polarity of the α and β heme pockets by using same-size isosteric mutations and obtained three mutant Hbs with a range of oxygen affinities.

In the β-chains, the authors replaced Leu^{28} (B10) with one asparagine βL^{28}(B10)N.[40] The oxygen-binding curves indicated that this mutant has an increase in oxygen affinity ($P_{50} \approx 1$ Torr) with respect to HbA ($P_{50} = 6.5$ Torr). This increase is probably due to an H-bond formation with bound oxygen that, by destabilizing the T-state, increases the oxygen affinity. This rHb was poorly expressed and unstable, thus a more complete characterization was not performed.

The authors replaced valine with threonine at position E11 in the E-helix of the α or β-chains.[41] The mutant, βV^{67}(E11)T, has a twofold decrease in oxygen affinity ($P_{50} = 12$ Torr) with respect to HbA ($P_{50} = 6.5$ Torr), and it retains a high level of cooperativity ($n = 2.2$ versus 2.6 in HbA). Crystallographic analysis indicated the presence of only subtle changes in the local geometry, with the presence of an H-bond between the O^{γ} atom of βV^{67}(E11)T and the backbone carbonyl of βHis^{63}(E7).[42] A water molecule, normally present in the heme pocket of Mb and α-chains but not in the β-chains, was not introduced as a result of this mutation. When this mutation was introduced at position Val^{62}(E11) of the α-chains, the functional effects were amplified and the oxygen affinity of αV^{62}(E11)T was decreased fourfold ($P_{50} = 25$ Torr), but cooperativity was practically absent ($n \approx 1.1$).[40] The significant decrease in oxygen affinity was attributed to stabilization of the water molecule present in the distal heme pocket, which becomes H-bonded to N^{ϵ} of αHis^{58}E7 and O^{γ} of αThr^{62}E11; in fact, this water molecule must be dissociated before oxygen bonding to the Fe-heme can take place.[40] The oxygen affinity and auto-oxidation rates of these heme-pocket mutants plus a surface mutant described below are compared in **Fig. 1A, B**. The efficiency of heme-pocket mutations for obtaining rHbs with varying oxygen affinities between ≈ 1.0 and 26 Torr is displayed in **Fig. 1A**. **Fig. 1B** shows that the decrease in oxygen affinity of αV^{62}(E11)T and βV^{67}(E11)T is accompanied by an increase in the auto-oxidation rates. Although this trend for increased auto-oxidation is usually associated with a decrease in oxygen affinity, increased auto-oxidation is, nevertheless, an unfavorable property for an HBOC.

A major obstacle to the development of HBOCs has been the appearance of peripheral vasoconstriction following infusion of some HBOCs.[8,43,44] NO depletion following extravasation of Hb is considered a major determinant of this negative phenomenon. An approach developed for preventing this effect is to hinder NO binding by introducing large aromatic or aliphatic groups to fill the proximal space of the heme pocket and decrease the free space available for NO binding to deoxygenated and oxygenated forms of Hb and, consequently, decrease the associated NO-dependent oxidation.[45] Several rHbs have been constructed to manipulate NO affinity. To the genetically α-α–cross-linked rHb1.1, the mutations $\alpha HisE7 \rightarrow$ Glu, $\alpha LeuB10 \rightarrow$ Trp, and $\beta ValE11 \rightarrow$ Trp have been introduced.[46] The pressor response was decreased in rats that were injected with this rHb with decreased NO affinity. This work implicates the importance of NO depletion in causing vasoconstriction. The authors also indicate

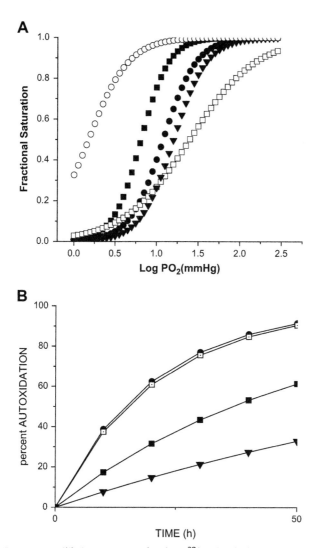

Fig. 1. (*A*) Oxygen equilibrium curves of rHb βL²⁸(B10)N (○), natural HbA (■) and rHbs βV⁶⁷(E11)T (●), αV⁶²(E11)T (□), and β(V1M + H2$_{deleted}$ + T4I + P5A + V76K) (▼). Measurements were performed in a phosphate buffer of 0.1 M at pH 7.4 and a temperature of 25°C. (*B*) Simulated auto-oxidation rates of HbA (■) and rHbs βV⁶⁷(E11)T (●), αV⁶²(E11)T (□), and β(V1M + H2$_{deleted}$ + T4I + P5A + V76K) (▼). Simulated T$_{1/2}$ of α-chain and β-chain auto-oxidation as calculated from data in Fronticelli C, Bellelli A, Brinigar WS. Approaches to the engineering of hemoglobin-based oxygen carriers. Transfusion Alternatives in Transfusion Medicine 2004; 5:516–522. The data indicate a twofold increase in the auto-oxidation in αV⁶²(E11)T and βV⁶⁷(E11)T with respect to HbA. Conversely, the auto-oxidation rate of the surface mutant β(V1M + H2$_{deleted}$ + T4I + P5A + V76K) was decreased threefold. Measurements were performed in a phosphate buffer of 0.1 M at pH 7.0 plus 1 mM ethylenediaminetetraacetate at a protein concentration of 60 μM in heme at a temperature of 37°C.

that vasoconstriction cannot be caused by excessive oxygen delivery[47] because the same vasoactivity was obtained by injecting rHb with a P_{50} of 30 Torr and 3 Torr. This conclusion, however, was based on the assumption that oxygen was not released by high-affinity HBOC, which may not be completely valid.[13,48,49]

The remaining question of whether it was possible to modify NO scavenging properties without modifying oxygen delivery capacity was tested using a mutant carrying heme-pocket modifications (details of which were not reported).[50,51] This rHb, denoted rHb 2.0 by Somatogen/Baxter, has a 20 to 30 fold decrease in NO affinity, a P_{50} of ≈ 30.0 Torr, and is polymerized by nondefined PEG treatment. It reduced pulmonary vasoconstrictive responses in isolated perfused rat lungs and improved intestinal oxygen delivery after hemorrhagic shock, as compared with rHb 1.1, which is a nondissociable tetrameric rHb with normally high NO affinity. These results support the proposition that it is possible to modify NO scavenging properties without impairing oxygen delivery. On the other hand, the combination of heme-pocket mutations, which hinder NO binding, and PEG polymerization, which hinders endothelial extravasation and associated NO depletion, may complicate the interpretation of comparison with a tetrameric rHb. Molecular size and oxygen affinity may play more important roles in the vasoconstrictor response to HBOC.[20,47]

SURFACE MUTATIONS

The optimal P_{50} for an HBOC is still under discussion. Earlier views were that an HBOC should have the same P_{50} as that of blood, and considerable efforts were devoted to the construction of rHbs with a high P_{50}. It is reasonable to expect that different clinical applications require HBOCs with different oxygen affinities. Low oxygen affinity is often correlated with a high auto-oxidation rate, and transfusion with a low-affinity Hb may pose a problem because the reduction systems in the plasma may not be sufficient to reduce the excessive reactive oxygen species that are produced by injection of large quantities of acellular Hb, with consequent endothelial damage and Hb extravasation.

The authors have constructed a human Hb with an intrinsically low oxygen affinity in the absence of heme pocket modifications. The amino acid substitutions introduced were $\beta(V1M + H2_{deleted} + T4I + P5A + V76K)$.[52,53] These mutations stabilize the low-oxygen-affinity conformation of HbA by increasing the hydrophobic interactions between the A-helix and the hydrophobic core of the β-subunits, thus mimicking the conformational effect of 2,3diphosphoglycerate interaction within the erythrocytes. In the presence of the Cl^- concentration in plasma (≈ 100–120 mM), the oxygen affinity of this rHb is similar to that of blood and cooperativity is retained. As shown in **Fig. 1**A, B, a positive aspect of this system of oxygen-affinity control is that the low oxygen affinity is associated with a decreased rate of auto-oxidation—approximately threefold lower than that of HbA—in contrast with the increased auto-oxidation rates seen with other low-affinity mutants.

Modification in oxygen affinity can also be obtained through substitutions at the subunit interfaces. These interfaces direct the Hb allosteric transition; thus, appropriate mutations can be introduced for modifying the equilibrium between R and T states of the molecule. The identification of nuclear magnetic resonance linked to the R-T transition has been especially important for the understanding of the conformational, dynamic, and functional properties of the Hb molecule. Stabilization of the T-structure results in an Hb with decreased oxygen affinity. Several Hbs with an oxygen affinity lower than that of HbA have been constructed.[54] An interesting mutant with favorable HBOC properties is $\beta N128Q + \alpha L29F$; it has an oxygen affinity similar to that of HbA, a 20 fold decrease in the NO-induced oxidation, and a reduced hypertensive effect on injection.

HEMOGLOBIN POLYMERIZATION

Another approach for inhibiting vasoconstriction associated with infusion of acellular heme protein is to construct polymerized Hb of large molecular mass to reduce the rate of extravasation through the endothelium. Native human and bovine Hbs have been polymerized by intra- and intermolecular chemical crosslinking.[15,18,20,55] Alternatively, the molecular volume has been increased by conjugation with PEG molecules.[21,56] Using genetic engineering, polymerization in the absence of chemical modification can be obtained by intermolecular disulfide (S-S) bond formation between cysteine residues introduced at favorable surface sites. Based on the model of the naturally occurring Hb Porto Alegre (βSer9 → Cys), polymerization has been obtained by introducing a cysteine at position β9. The authors developed three different polymeric rHbs: Hb Prisca, Hb Polytaur, and Hb (Polytaur)$_n$.[36,57,58]

In Hb Prisca, β(S9C + C93A + C112G), the naturally occurring β93Cys and β112Cys of HbA were replaced by alanine and glycine, respectively, to prevent the formation of spurious S-S bonds during the refolding, and doing so restricted polymerization to β9 cysteine.[57] The β9Cys residues are pointed toward the solvent in a favorable reacting position. The angle measured between the Cα of the two β9 residues with respect to the geometric center of the HbA tetramer is 108.4 degrees. This geometry introduces steric hindrance that limits the extent of polymerization from 7 to 8 tetrameric Hb molecules, which were tightly packed and assembled into a globular shape. The mutations that were introduced and the polymerization reaction did not alter the functional characteristics of Hb Prisca, that is, oxygen affinity, stability to denaturation, and auto-oxidation remained similar to that of natural HbA.

As mentioned, the hybrid Hb molecule Hb Minotaur has a high expression yield and is expressed in tetrameric soluble form in *Escherichia coli*.[36] Introduction into Hb Minotaur of the same substitution that is present in Hb Prisca produces a polymeric rHb composed of 7–8 tetrameric Hb molecules (MW $\approx$ 500kD). The authors refer to this polymer as Hb Polytaur.[36] This process is slow ($\approx$ 4 weeks), probably due to the slow kinetics of tetrameric molecule incorporation into a globular polymeric species. Polymerization did not modify the oxygen affinity, which remained similar to that of HbA (17 Torr at 37°C). The rate of heme release, which is indicative of the stability of the protein, showed a tenfold increase in heme affinity as compared with that of HbA.[36,40] Measurements of auto-oxidation rates in whole blood at 37°C gave a half-time ($T_{1/2}$) of 46 hours, well compatible with the 20–36 hour $T_{1/2}$ retention time in circulation that has been measured in humans using other polymerized Hbs.[16,59,60] Because polymerization was obtained by formation of S-S bonds, the authors determined the stability of the polymer toward the reducing agents present in the blood. Polymerization, as determined by size-exclusion chromatography, was not altered. The S-S bonds are $\approx$ 2.4 Å long, and their accessibility to reducing agents is probably hindered by the numerous interactions that result from the intermolecular cross-linking of the subunits. In **Fig. 2**, the $T_{1/2}$ of intravascular retention of polymeric Hb in human (36 hours) is compared with the $T_{1/2}$ of auto-oxidation (46 hours) and with heme loss (10-fold slower than for natural HbA). The graph illustrates that the rates of auto-oxidation and heme loss are slower than the clearance from the circulation. As discussed later, transfusion of this polymer was not associated with an increase in arterial pressure and is most effective in reducing cerebral ischemia. The authors conclude that Hb Polytaur has the desirable characteristics of an HBOC.

When the cysteine residues were introduced at position β9 without the substitution of the natural cysteines, a rapid polymerization occurred in less than 1 hour.[40,58] The authors refer to this polymer as Hb (Polytaur)$_n$. This polymer has a heterogeneous

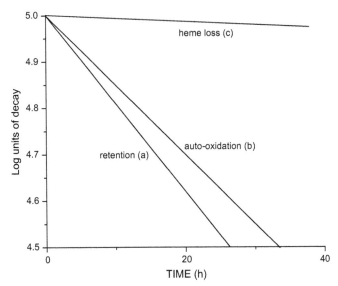

Fig. 2. Semilogarithmic plots of the retention time in circulation of (a) polymeric Hb concentration in humans simulated from the $T_{1/2}$ data, (b) the residual oxygenated form, simulated from the $T_{1/2}$ of the auto-oxidation rate in whole blood at 37°C, and (c) the empiric representation of heme affinity of Hb Polytaur, at least 10 fold that of HbA. The data indicate that the conformational stability of Hb Polytaur, as determined by the values of auto-oxidation in whole blood and of heme affinity, is well within the limits of retention time of polymeric hemoglobin in the circulation. Simulation for (a) was based on data from Refs. [59,16,60]. Simulation for (b) and (c) was based on data from Bobofchak KM, Mito T, Texel SJ, et al. A recombinant polymeric hemoglobin with conformational, functional, and physiological characteristics of an in vivo O_2 transporter. Am J Physiol Heart Circ Physiol 2003;285:H549–61; and Fronticelli C, Bellelli A, Brinigar WS. Approaches to the engineering of hemoglobin-based oxygen carriers. Trans Alt in Trans Med 2004;5:516–20.

molecular weight, with the main species having a molecular weight of 1000 kDa and higher. Oxygen-binding measurements indicated that Hb (Polytaur)$_n$ has oxygen-binding characteristics similar to Mb, that is, high oxygen affinity (P_{50} = ≈2.0 Torr) and absent (loss) of cooperativity (n = 1). The affinity for heme remained high, but the auto-oxidation rate, although not directly measured, seemed to be increased with respect to Hb Polytaur. These properties are similar to those of ZL-HbBv,[20] wherein polymerization occurs at sporadic loci. Therefore, directing the sites of polymerization specifically at the β9 cysteine residue in Hb Polytaur permits interactions among subunits in the tetramer to be retained and oxygen affinity to remain similar to that of acellular HbA.

A polymer of two tetrameric Hb molecules (MW 130kD) has been obtained by introducing in the human β-chains a Cys residue at position β83, replacing a Gly residue.[61] This polymer has an auto-oxidation rate similar to that of HbA, stability toward the reducing agents present in blood, an oxygen affinity similar to that of HbA, and a high degree of size homogeneity and stability, and it does not dissociate into smaller species. Addition of a second mutation, F41Y, has been found to further decrease the oxygen affinity of this polymer.

HEMOGLOBIN-INDUCED ENDOTHELIAL PERMEABILITY

The negative effects of HBOC infusion are to a great extent correlated with their endo-thelial permeability due to the production of reactive oxygen species.[4,62] The authors addressed this problem by investigating the effect of HbA and the two polymerized Hbs on the integrity of bovine lung microvascular endothelial cell monolayers to have a quantitative assessment of the rate of Hb extravasation and Hb-induced permeability.[63] Hb flux through the monolayer was directly linked to the size of each Hb molecule, thereby demonstrating the ability of the endothelial cell monolayer to sieve the three Hb species. Calculation of the diffusive permeability coefficients over the 4-hour observation showed that the increase in the diffusive permeability in the three systems is directly correlated to their diffusion coefficient, indicating the potentiality of Hb molecules to induce damage of the monolayer endothelium with formation of gaps, through which the diffusion of Hb is a function of the molecular mass and the hydrodynamic radius of the protein.

In vivo, acellular Hb was also capable of opening endothelial pores in the intestinal microcirculation. However, the number of albumin leakage sites was much greater with α–α–cross-linked tetrameric Hb transfusion than with polymeric Hb or PEG-Hb transfusion.[62,64] Thus, the endothelium appears to be more resistant to damage from the larger polymeric Hb and PEG-Hb in vivo than in vitro. The increased leakage was attributed to NO depletion, degranulation of mast cells, and histamine release.[62,65,66] Permeability data with rHb are more limited. In isolated rat lung, neither stabilized tetrameric rHb nor pegylated rHb with low NO affinity increased the capillary filtration coefficient for water flux.[50] Therefore, more work is necessary to understand the mechanisms of increased intestinal endothelial permeability by acellular Hb, whether similar mechanisms are activated in other vascular beds, and whether these mechanisms are also activated by the various rHbs.

RECOMBINANT HEMOGLOBIN AND OXYGEN DELIVERY

The amount of rHb produced with the authors' *Escherichia coli* expression system permitted in vivo evaluation in mice. Hypervolemic exchange transfusion of an Hb Pol-ytaur solution produced a small increase in arterial pressure that was (a) similar to that produced by hypervolemic exchange transfusion of an albumin solution and (b) less than the increase produced by transfusion of cross-linked Hb solution.[36] Transfusion of cross-linked tetrameric Hb is known to produce hypertension that is related to scav-enging of NO surrounding the vascular smooth muscle and is thought to be related to extravasation in vascular beds with large endothelial pores. The similar changes in arterial pressure that occurred with Hb Polytaur and albumin transfusion suggest that the primary reason for the observed hypertension was volume expansion rather than excessive scavenging of NO. Thus, this polymer of 7–8 tetramers appears to be of sufficient size to limit extravasation and scavenging of vascular NO.

The ability of high-oxygen-affinity Hb polymers to deliver oxygen to ischemic tissue was assessed in experimental stroke.[36,58,67] In mice subjected to transient occlusion of the middle cerebral artery, collateral arteries maintained residual blood flow at $\approx 20\%$ of normal in the ischemic core and at intermediate levels in the border regions. Exchange transfusion with acellular Hb permitted hematocrit and blood viscosity to be reduced without a large decrease in oxygen-carrying capacity. **Fig. 3** compares infarct volumes after 2 hours of occlusion in mice that underwent hypervolemic exchange transfusion of various solutions starting at 10 minutes of occlusion. Data were compiled from experiments with Hb Polytaur, Hb (Polytaur)$_n$, and bovine Hb that was chemically polymerized without the polymerization chemicals remaining on the

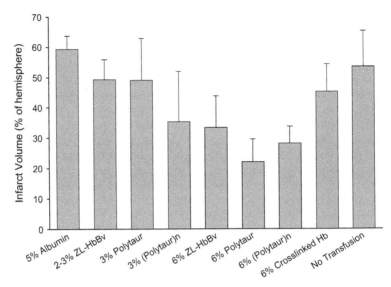

Fig. 3. Brain infarct volume expressed as a percent of cerebral hemisphere (mean ± SD) in mice subjected to 2 hours of transient occlusion of the middle cerebral artery. At 10 minutes of focal cerebral ischemia, a hypervolemic exchange transfusion was performed in which 0.95 mL of various solutions was infused and 0.7 mL of blood was withdrawn. *(Data from Nemoto M, Mito T, Brinigar WS, et al. Salvage of focal cerebral ischemic damage by transfusion of high O_2-affinity recombinant hemoglobin polymers in mouse. J Appl Phys 2006; 100:1688–91; and Mito T, Nemoto M, Kwansa H, et al. Decreased damage from transient focal cerebral ischemia by transfusion of zero-link hemoglobin polymers in mouse. Stroke 2009;40:278–84.)*

polymer (zero-link bovine Hb; ZL-HbBv).[36,58,67] The latter has a low P_{50} (3–4 Torr) that is comparable to that of Hb (Polytaur)$_n$ (2–3 Torr). When transfused at a concentration of ≈3%, infarct volume was decreased most effectively by the Hb (Polytaur)$_n$, compared with a group transfused with a 5% solution of albumin. At a 6% concentration, the reduction in infarct size became more prominent with ZL-HbBv. Hb Polytaur with a P_{50} of 17 Torr was the most effective polymer at the 6% concentration. By comparison, exchange transfusion of a 6% solution of sebacoyl–cross-linked tetrameric Hb with a P_{50} of 34 Torr[68] produced only a marginal decrease in infarct volume. Together, these data indicate that acellular Hb with a P_{50} below that of RBC-based Hb can rescue tissue from ischemic stroke. Furthermore, the data support the notion that the properties of an HBOC can be tailored to a specific clinical use.

Intraischemic oxygen transport by an HBOC can be influenced by several biophysical factors. A low-P_{50} HBOC will act to limit precapillary oxygen loss and unload a greater proportion of its oxygen in the low-oxygen environment of ischemic tissue. Although a high P_{50} of RBC-based Hb can be beneficial in ischemic stroke models,[69] the high P_{50} of RBC-based Hb enables the PO_2 gradient between the RBC and endothelium to be increased and helps to overcome the considerable resistance to overall oxygen transport within plasma. With Hb present in the plasma space, the solubility of oxygen in plasma is increased, and the resistance to oxygen diffusion throughout the plasma is effectively decreased.[9,10] Consequently, an HBOC with a P_{50} that is between the P_{50} of RBC-based Hb and the tissue PO_2 may facilitate the diffusion of oxygen from the RBC to the endothelial wall. Another factor to consider is that RBCs form a single line in capillaries and are interspersed with plasma. During incomplete ischemia, RBCs move at a sluggish pace and their velocity and numbers per capillary become highly heterogeneous. By decreasing hematocrit with an exchange transfusion, velocity should be increased. By having an HBOC in the plasma, the effective surface area for oxygen diffusion increases. The net result is likely to be an increase in the homogeneity of oxygen flux. Thus, several theoretical mechanisms should promote oxygen delivery by acellular Hb during ischemic stroke.

MYOGLOBIN AS OXYGEN TRANSPORTER AND PLASMA EXPANDER

Mb is a monomeric protein present in striated muscle that has been extensively studied; it was the first protein structure determined at high resolution by x-ray crystallography and is a model system for many heme protein studies. The soluble holoprotein is expressed in *Escherichia coli*.[70] Recombinant Mb (rMb) has the conformational and functional characteristics of the native protein.

Because high-oxygen-affinity HBOCs appear to be effective in delivering oxygen, it is conceivable that rMb could be designed as an efficient oxygen carrier, provided that it does not extravasate. To this end, genetic engineering can be applied to construct Mb systems endowed with a large molecular mass. Moreover, Mb has been the model system in the design of Hb with reduced NO scavenging properties.[37] Polymerization of the monomeric Mb is obtained on the same principle used for Hb polymerization.[36,40] The authors observed that in sperm whale Mb, in which cysteine residues are absent, the introduction of the substitutions Gln8 → Cys, Lys50 → Cys, and Lys76 → Cys results in the formation of a large polymeric species with molecular weights between 25 and 1000 kDa. On oxidation with ferricyanide, the polymerization is essentially instantaneous. Filtration of the polymerized Mb through a Sephadex column in which a small volume of a dithionite solution has been layered on the top reduces the Mb to its ferrous state without affecting its polymerization characteristics.

Mb molecules could also be chemically modified by alkylation of the lysine residues with PEG. Alternatively, Mb mutants in which one or more cysteine residues have been introduced could be specifically modified by reaction with maleimide-PEG.[71] In both cases, the final results would be a Mb molecule with a large hydrodynamic volume, plasma expander properties, and oxygen delivery capacity.

SUMMARY

Using recombinant technology, it is possible to modulate the functional characteristics of the Hb molecule and produce Hbs to be used as resuscitating fluids in different therapeutic applications. Heme-pocket substitutions can be used to modulate oxygen affinity and to hinder NO depletion and the associated vasoconstriction. Alternatively, surface mutations are also effective in decreasing oxygen affinity in the absence of increased auto-oxidation rate. Polymerization by intermolecular S-S cross-links can be used to produce a homogeneous globular polymer that has an auto-oxidation rate and conformational stability in vivo that are well compatible with the retention time in circulation of polymerized Hbs in human. Transfusion of polymerized mutant Hbs with a P_{50} below that of RBC Hb is capable of reducing brain ischemic injury, thereby indicating that these high-oxygen-affinity rHbs may be useful in the treatment of a variety of clinical conditions of oxygen deprivation. In conclusion, recombinant technology allows the design of a variety of Hbs with HBOC potential. However, a large production capacity of rHb for widespread clinical use as a general blood substitute is at present difficult to achieve and remains the crucial challenge.

ACKNOWLEDGMENTS

The authors are grateful to Tzipora Sofare, MA, for her editorial assistance.

REFERENCES

1. Baron JF. Blood substitutes. Haemoglobin therapeutics in clinical practice. Crit Care 1999;3:R99–102.
2. Chang TM. Red blood cell substitutes. Baillieres Best Pract Res Clin Haematol 2000;13:651–67.
3. Stowell CP, Levin J, Spiess BD, et al. Progress in the development of RBC substitutes. Transfusion 2001;41:287–99.
4. Alayash AI. Oxygen therapeutics: can we tame haemoglobin? Nat Rev Drug Discov 2004;3:152–9.
5. Stowell C. Blood substitutes: time for a deep breath. Transfusion 2008;48:574–5.
6. Urbaitis B, Razynska A, Corteza Q, et al. Intravascular retention and renal handling of purified natural and intramolecularly cross-linked hemoglobins. J Lab Clin Med 1991;117:115–21.
7. Matheson B, Razynska A, Kwansa H, et al. Appearance of dissociable and cross-linked hemoglobins in the renal hilar lymph. J Lab Clin Med 2000;135:459–64.
8. Sampei K, Ulatowski JA, Asano Y, et al. Role of nitric oxide scavenging in vascular response to cell-free hemoglobin transfusion. Am J Physiol Heart Circ Physiol 2005;289:H1191–201.
9. Page TC, Light WR, McKay CB, et al. Oxygen transport by erythrocyte/hemoglobin solution mixtures in an in vitro capillary as a model of hemoglobin-based oxygen carrier performance. Microvasc Res 1998;55:54–64.
10. McCarthy MR, Vandegriff KD, Winslow RM. The role of facilitated diffusion in oxygen transport by cell-free hemoglobins: implications for the design of hemoglobin-based oxygen carriers. Biophys Chem 2001;92:103–17.
11. Winslow RM. Targeted O_2 delivery by low-p50 hemoglobin: a new basis for hemoglobin-based oxygen carriers. Artif Cells Blood Substit Immobil Biotechnol 2005; 33:1–12.
12. Tsai AG, Cabrales P, Manjula BN, et al. Dissociation of local nitric oxide concentration and vasoconstriction in the presence of cell-free hemoglobin oxygen carriers. Blood 2006;108:3603–10.
13. Tsai AG, Vandegriff KD, Intaglietta M, et al. Targeted O_2 delivery by low-P50 hemoglobin: a new basis for O_2 therapeutics. Am J Physiol Heart Circ Physiol 2003;285:H1411–9.
14. Wettstein R, Tsai AG, Erni D, et al. Resuscitation with polyethylene glycol–modified human hemoglobin improves microcirculatory blood flow and tissue oxygenation after hemorrhagic shock in awake hamsters. Crit Care Med 2003;31: 1824–30.
15. Winslow RM. $\alpha\alpha$-crosslinked hemoglobin: was failure predicted by preclinical testing? Vox Sang 2000;79:1–20.
16. Hughes GS, Antal EJ, Locker PK, et al. Physiology and pharmacokinetics of a novel hemoglobin-based oxygen carrier in humans. Crit Care Clin 1996;24: 756–64.
17. Kasper SM, Walter M, Grune F, et al. Effects of a hemoglobin-based oxygen carrier (HBOC-201) on hemodynamics and oxygen transport in patients

undergoing preoperative hemodilution for elective abdominal aortic surgery. Anesth Analg 1996;83:921–7.

18. Gould SA, Moore EE, Hoyt DB, et al. The first randomized trial of human polymerized hemoglobin as a blood substitute in acute trauma and emergent surgery. J Am Coll Surg 1998;187:113–20.

19. Gould SA, Moore EE, Hoyt DB, et al. The life-sustaining capacity of human polymerized hemoglobin when red cells might be unavailable. J Am Coll Surg 2002; 195:445–52.

20. Matheson B, Kwansa HE, Bucci E, et al. Vascular response to infusions of a non-extravasating hemoglobin polymer. J Appl Phys 2002;93:1479–86.

21. Nho K, Glower D, Bredehoeft S, et al. PEG-bovine hemoglobin: safety in a canine dehydrated hypovolemic-hemorrhagic shock model. Biomater Artif Cells Immobilization Biotechnol 1992;20:511–24.

22. Olofsson C, Ahl T, Johansson T, et al. A multicenter clinical study of the safety and activity of maleimide-polyethylene glycol-modified hemoglobin (Hemospan) in patients undergoing major orthopedic surgery. Anesthesiology 2006;105: 1153–63.

23. Olofsson C, Nygards EB, Ponzer S, et al. A randomized, single-blind, increasing dose safety trial of an oxygen-carrying plasma expander (Hemospan) administered to orthopaedic surgery patients with spinal anaesthesia. Transfus Med 2008;18:28–39.

24. Natanson C, Kern SJ, Lurie P, et al. Cell-free hemoglobin-based blood substitutes and risk of myocardial infarction and death: a meta-analysis. JAMA 2008;299:2304–12.

25. Nagai K, Thogersen HC. Generation of beta-globin by sequence-specific proteolysis of a hybrid protein produced in Escherichia coli. Nature 1984;309:810–2.

26. Fronticelli C, O'Donnell JK, Brinigar WS. Recombinant human hemoglobin: expression and refolding of beta-globin from Escherichia coli. J Protein Chem 1991;10:495–501.

27. Tame J, Shih DT, Pagnier J, et al. Functional role of the distal valine (E11) residue of alpha subunits in human haemoglobin. J Mol Biol 1991;218:761–7.

28. Sanna MT, Razynska A, Karavitis M, et al. Assembly of human hemoglobin. Studies with Escherichia coli–expressed alpha-globin. J Biol Chem 1997;272:3478–86.

29. Looker D, Abbott-Brown D, Cozart P, et al. A human recombinant haemoglobin designed for use as a blood substitute. Nature 1992;356:258–60.

30. Looker D, Mathews AJ, Neway JO, et al. Expression of recombinant human hemoglobin in Escherichia coli. Meth Enzymol 1994;231:364–74.

31. Shen TJ, Ho NT, Simplaceanu V, et al. Production of unmodified human adult hemoglobin in Escherichia coli. Proc Natl Acad Sci USA 1993;90:8108–12.

32. Scott EE, Paster EV, Olson JS. The stabilities of mammalian apomyoglobins vary over a 600-fold range and can be enhanced by comparative mutagenesis. J Biol Chem 2000;275:27129–36.

33. Kihm AJ, Kong Y, Hong W, et al. An abundant erythroid protein that stabilizes free alpha-haemoglobin. Nature 2002;417:758–63.

34. Gell D, Kong Y, Eaton SA, et al. Biophysical characterization of the alpha-globin binding protein alpha-hemoglobin stabilizing protein. J Biol Chem 2002;277: 40602–9.

35. Feng L, Gell DA, Zhou S, et al. Molecular mechanism of AHSP-mediated stabilization of alpha-hemoglobin. Cell 2004;119:629–40.

36. Bobofchak KM, Mito T, Texel SJ, et al. A recombinant polymeric hemoglobin with conformational, functional, and physiological characteristics of an in vivo O_2 transporter. Am J Physiol Heart Circ Physiol 2003;285:H549–61.

37. Olson JS. Genetic engineering of myoglobin as a simple prototype for hemo-globin-based blood substitutes. Artif Cells Blood Substit Immobil Biotechnol 1994;22:429–41.
38. Springer BA, Sligar SG, Olson JS, et al. Mechanisms of ligand recognition by myoglobin. Chem Rev 1994;94:699–714.
39. Piro MC, Militello V, Leone M, et al. Heme pocket disorder in myoglobin: reversal by acid-induced soft refolding. Biochemistry 2001;40:11841–50.
40. Fronticelli C, Bellelli A, Brinigar WS. Approaches to the engineering of hemo-globin-based oxygen carriers. Transfus Altern Transfus Med 2004;5:516–22.
41. Fronticelli C, Brinigar WS, Olson JS, et al. Recombinant human hemoglobin: modification of the polarity of the beta-heme pocket by a valine67(E11)→threo-nine mutation. Biochemistry 1993;32:1235–42.
42. Pechik I, Ji X, Fidelis K, et al. Crystallographic, molecular modeling, and biophys-ical characterization of the valine beta 67 (E11)→threonine variant of hemo-globin. Biochemistry 1996;35:1935–45.
43. Olson JS, Foley EW, Rogge C, et al. NO scavenging and the hypertensive effect of hemoglobin-based blood substitutes. Free Radic Biol Med 2004;36:685–97.
44. Ulatowski JA, Nishikawa T, Matheson-Urbaitis B, et al. Regional blood flow alter-ations after bovine fumaryl ββ–crosslinked hemoglobin transfusion and nitric oxide synthase inhibition. Crit Care Med 1996;24:558–65.
45. Olson JS, Maillett DS. Designing recombinant hemoglobin for use as a blood substitute. In: Winslow RM, editor. Blood substitutes. Amsterdam: Academic Press/Elsevier; 2006. p. 354–74.
46. Doherty DH, Doyle MP, Curry SR, et al. Rate of reaction with nitric oxide determines the hypertensive effect of cell-free hemoglobin. Nat Biotechnol 1998;16:672–6.
47. Rohlfs RJ, Bruner E, Chiu A, et al. Arterial blood pressure responses to cell-free hemoglobin solutions and the reaction with nitric oxide. J Biol Chem 1998;273: 12128–34.
48. Qin X, Kwansa H, Bucci E, et al. Role of 20-HETE in the pial arteriolar constrictor response to decreased hematocrit after exchange transfusion of cell-free polymeric hemoglobin. J Appl Phys 2006;100:336–42.
49. Koehler RC, Fronticelli C, Bucci E. Insensitivity of cerebral oxygen transport to oxygen affinity of hemoglobin-based oxygen carriers. Biochim Biophys Acta 2008;1784:1387–94.
50. Resta TC, Walker BR, Eichinger MR, et al. Rate of NO scavenging alters effects of recombinant hemoglobin solutions on pulmonary vasoreactivity. J Appl Phys 2002;93:1327–36.
51. Raat NJ, Liu JF, Doyle MP, et al. Effects of recombinant-hemoglobin solutions rHb2.0 and rHb1.1 on blood pressure, intestinal blood flow, and gut oxygenation in a rat model of hemorrhagic shock. J Lab Clin Med 2005;145:21–32.
52. Fronticelli C, Sanna MT, Perez-Alvarado GC, et al. Allosteric modulation by tertiary structure in mammalian hemoglobins. Introduction of the functional char-acteristics of bovine hemoglobin into human hemoglobin by five amino acid substitutions. J Biol Chem 1995;270:30588–92.
53. Fronticelli C, Bobofchak KM, Karavitis M, et al. Introduction of a new regulatory mechanism into human hemoglobin. Biophys Chem 2002;98:115–26.
54. Tsai CH, Ho C. Recombinant hemoglobins with low oxygen affinity and high cooperativity. Biophys Chem 2002;98:15–25.
55. Pearce L, Gawryl M. Overview of preclinical and clinical efficacy of Biopure's HBOCs. In: Chang T, editor. Blood substitutes: principles, methods, products and clinical trials. Basel (Switzerland): Karger/Landes; 1998.

56. Svergun DI, Ekstrom F, Vandegriff KD, et al. Solution structure of poly (ethylene) glycol–conjugated hemoglobin revealed by small-angle X-ray scattering: implications for a new oxygen therapeutic. Biophys J 2008;94:173–81.
57. Fronticelli C, Arosio D, Bobofchak KM, et al. Molecular engineering of a polymer of tetrameric hemoglobins. Proteins 2001;44:212–22.
58. Nemoto M, Mito T, Brinigar WS, et al. Salvage of focal cerebral ischemic damage by transfusion of high O_2-affinity recombinant hemoglobin polymers in mouse. J Appl Phys 2006;100:1688–91.
59. Hughes GS, Francom SF, Antal EJ, et al. Hematologic effects of a novel hemoglobin-based oxygen carrier in normal male and female subjects. J Lab Clin Med 1995;126:444–51.
60. Carmichael FJ, Ali AC, Campbell JA, et al. A phase I study of oxidized raffinose cross-linked human hemoglobin. Crit Care Med 2000;28:2283–92.
61. Fablet C, Marden MC, Green BN, et al. Stable octameric structure of recombinant hemoglobin alpha(2)beta(2)83 Gly→Cys. Protein Sci 2003;12:690–5.
62. Baldwin AL. Modified hemoglobins produce venular interendothelial gaps and albumin leakage in the rat mesentery. Am J Phys 1999;277:H650–9.
63. Dull RO, DeWitt BJ, Dinavahi R, et al. Quantitative assessment of hemoglobin-induced endothelial barrier dysfunction. J Appl Phys 2004;97:1930–7.
64. Baldwin AL, Wiley EB, Alayash AI. Comparison of effects of two hemoglobin-based O_2 carriers on intestinal integrity and microvascular leakage. Am J Physiol Heart Circ Physiol 2002;283:H1292–301.
65. Baldwin AL, Wilson LM, Valeski JE. Ultrastructural effects of intravascularly injected polyethylene glycol–hemoglobin in intestinal mucosa. Am J Physiol Heart Circ Physiol 1998;275:H615–25.
66. Burke TK, Teng X, Patel RP, et al. Effects of S-nitrosation on hemoglobin-induced microvascular damage. Antioxid Redox Signal 2006;8:1093–101.
67. Mito T, Nemoto M, Kwansa H, et al. Decreased damage from transient focal cerebral ischemia by transfusion of zero-link hemoglobin polymers in mouse. Stroke 2009;40:278–84.
68. Bucci E, Razynska A, Kwansa H, et al. Production and characteristics of an infusible oxygen-carrying fluid based on hemoglobin intramolecularly cross-linked with sebacic acid. J Lab Clin Med 1996;128:146–53.
69. Watson JC, Doppenberg EMR, Bullock MR, et al. Effects of the allosteric modification of hemoglobin on brain oxygen and infarct size in a feline model of stroke. Stroke 1997;28:1624–30.
70. Springer BA, Sligar SG. High-level expression of sperm whale myoglobin in E coli. Proc Natl Acad Sci USA 1987;84:8961–5.
71. Manjula BN, Tsai AG, Intaglietta M, et al. Conjugation of multiple copies of polyethylene glycol to hemoglobin facilitated through thiolation: influence on hemoglobin structure and function. Protein J 2005;24:133–46.

Nanobiotechnology for Hemoglobin-based Blood Substitutes

T.M.S. Chang, OC, MD, CM, PhD, FRCPC, FRS(C)

KEYWORDS

- Nanobiotechnology • Hemoglobin • Polyhemoglobin
- Catalase • Superoxide dismutase • Nanomedicine
- Blood substitutes • Fibrinogen • Tyrosinase • Melanoma

Nanobiotechnology is the assembling of biological molecules into 1- to 100-nanometer dimensions. These dimensions can be the diameter of nanodimensional artificial cells or particles, membranes with nanodimension thicknesses, or nanotubules with nanodimension diameters. The first nanobiotechnological approach reported in the literature was the cross-linking of hemoglobin (Hb) into ultrathin polyhemoglobin (polyHb) membranes for artificial red blood cell (RBC) membranes.[1,2] If the emulsion is made even smaller, then whole artificial cells with their Hb can be cross-linked into polyHb of the nanodimension. Glutaraldehyde can cross-link Hb into soluble polyHb of the nanodimension.[3] New generations of this approach include the nanobiotechnological assembly of Hb, catalase (CAT), and superoxide dismutase (SOD) into a soluble nano-dimension complex. This acts as an oxygen carrier and as an antioxidant for those conditions with potential for ischemia-reperfusion injuries.[4–7] Another recent novel approach is the assembling of Hb and fibrinogen into a soluble nanodimension polyHb-fibrinogen complex that acts as an oxygen carrier with platelet-like activity.[6] This is potentially useful in cases of extensive blood loss requiring massive replacement using blood substitutes, resulting in the need for replacement of platelets and clotting factors. Nanodimension artificial cells can also be formed as nanodimension biodegradable polymeric membrane artificial cells containing Hb and RBC enzymes.[4–6]

POLYHEMOGLOBIN
Basic Principles

Hb is a tetramer $(\alpha 1\beta 1\alpha 2\beta 2)^8$ that breaks down into toxic dimers $(\alpha 1\beta 1$ and $\alpha 2\beta 2)$ that cause vasoconstriction, renal toxicity, and other adverse effects. Even in the form of

The author acknowledges ongoing research grants from the Canadian Institutes of Health Research and the Quebec Ministry of Health's Hemovigilance Program in the form of funding for a FRSQ Research Group (d'equip) on Blood Substitutes in Transfusion Medicine.
Artificial Cells and Organs Research Center, McGill University, 3655 Drummond Street, Montreal, Quebec H3Y 1Y6, Canada
E-mail address: artcell.med@mcgill.ca

tetramers, Hb molecules can cross the intercellular junction of blood vessels to cause adverse vasopressor effects. The author used the principle of nanobiotechnology to assemble Hb molecules into nanodimension polyHb, first using the bifunctional agent sebacyl chloride,[1,2] then using glutaraldehyde.[3] The glutaraldehyde method was developed independently by other groups for the development of Hb-based oxygen carriers for clinical trials.[9,10]

Present Status of Polyhemoglobin in Clinical Trials

Phase III clinical trials have been completed on over 171 patients, showing that this product can successfully replace extensive blood loss in patients undergoing trauma surgery and other surgery by maintaining the total Hb level at the 8–10 g/dL range needed for safe surgery, with no reported side effects.[9] For example, transfusion of this polyHb in patients with Hb levels as low as 2 g/dL can raise the Hb level to within the 8 to 10 g/dL range, with the patients recovering from surgery. Normally, patients with Hb levels of less than 3 g/dL do not survive. Steven Gould (Northfield Co.) and colleagues have infused up to 10 L of polyHb into individual trauma-surgery patients. In the United States, this product has been approved for compassionate use in patients, and it is awaiting a regulatory decision for routine clinical uses. Gould and colleagues have performed Phase III clinical trials on its use in prehospital emergencies in which no typing and cross-matching is needed, so that it can be used right on the spot.[11]

Given that the supply of Hb from outdated donor blood is limited, a glutaraldehyde–cross-linked bovine polyHb has been developed and tested in phase III clinical trials.[10] For example, Pearce and colleagues in the United States have performed a multicenter, multinational, randomized, single-blind, RBC-controlled Phase III clinical trial in patients undergoing elective orthopedic surgery. A total of 688 patients were randomized in a 1:1 ratio to receive either the polyHb or RBCs at the time of the first perioperative RBC transfusion decision. Of the patients receiving polyHb, 59.4% required no RBC transfusion all the way to follow up, 96.3% avoided transfusion with RBCs on the first postoperative day, and up to 70.3% avoided RBC transfusion up to day 7 after surgery. In North America, this bovine polyHb has been approved for compassionate use in patients, and in South Africa, this product is approved for use in adult surgery patients to treat acute anemia and reduce allogeneic blood use.

Effects of Tetrameric Hemoglobin in Polyhemoglobin on Vasoconstriction and Adverse Cardiac Effects

In addition to the above two polyHbs (one from a human source, one from a bovine source), other modified Hbs have also been prepared and studied. These include intramolecularly cross-linked tetrameric Hb and polyHb containing more than 30% tetrameric Hb that can cause vasoconstriction. This has led to the proposal that the intercellular junctions of the endothelial lining of the vascular wall allow molecular dimension Hb to enter into the interstitial space. There, Hb acts as a sink in binding and removing nitric oxide needed for maintaining the normal tone of smooth muscles. This results in the constriction of blood vessels and other smooth muscles especially those of the esophagus and the gastrointestinal tract. To test this, the author and colleagues prepared polyHbs containing different percentages of unpolymerized Hb molecules using the same glutaraldehyde cross-link and characterized to ensure that they all have the same oxygen affinity.[12] The results show that the polyHb with the lowest percentage of unpolymerized Hb molecules does not cause vasoconstriction. With increasing percentages of unpolymerized Hb molecules, there are increasing degrees of vasoconstriction. Rats hearts have high heart rates and are therefore more sensitive to ischemic changes. Recent studies by the author and colleagues in rats show ischemic ECG changes in the form of ST elevation when rats received polyHb with a high percentage of tetrameric Hb. With even higher percentages of tetrameric Hb, there was ECG evidence of cardiac arrhythmia. ST elevation could be due to coronary vasoconstriction, resulting in a decrease in the supply of oxygen to the heart, and this may explain the observation of small subendocardial lesions in some primates and swine after infusion with one type of modified Hb consisting of 100% single-Hb molecules. Thus, to avoid causing adverse vasopressor or cardiac effects, polyHb preparations must contain less than 2% of tetrameric Hb.

NEW GENERATION OF NANOBIOTECHNOLOGY-BASED BLOOD SUBSTITUTES: ASSEMBLING HEMOGLOBIN WITH CATALASE AND SUPEROXIDE DISMUTASE
Rationale

PolyHb is likely to have an important role in certain clinical applications. However, for conditions with the potential for ischemia-reperfusion injuries, the use of a new generation of blood substitute that is an oxygen carrier and an antioxidant should be considered. The reasons for this are that a lack of oxygen supply in heart, sustained hemorrhagic shock, stroke, organ transplantation, and other conditions may result in ischemia. Ischemia leads to alterations in metabolic reactions, producing hypoxanthine and activating the enzyme xanthine oxidase. The level of hypoxanthine increases with the duration and severity of the ischemia. When the tissues are reperfused with oxygen-carrying fluid, xanthine oxidase converts oxygen and hypoxanthine into superoxide. By several mechanisms, superoxide results in the formation of oxygen radicals that can cause tissue injury.

Even in routine surgery, it will be important to rule out patients with cardiac ischemia when using modified Hb with no antioxidants. Otherwise, there could be adverse cardiac effects related to ischemia-reperfusion. Other conditions in which ischemia-reperfusion injuries would be likely include severe sustained hemorrhagic shock, stroke, myocardial infarction, and organ transplantation. For all of the above situations, the author and colleagues used nanobiotechnology to assemble Hb with CAT and SOD into soluble nanodimension polyHb-CAT-SOD (**Fig. 1**).[13] This is an oxygen carrier with the ability to remove oxygen radicals. SOD and CAT convert superoxide into hydrogen peroxide that is in turn converted into water and oxygen.

Compared with polyHb, polyHb-CAT-SOD removes significantly more oxygen radicals and peroxides and stabilizes the cross-linked Hb, resulting in a decrease in oxidative iron and heme release.[4–6] Cross-linking these enzymes to polyHb is important because otherwise free SOD and CAT are removed rapidly from the circulation, with a half-time of less than 30 minutes. In the form of polyHb-CAT-SOD, these enzymes circulate with a half-time more comparable with polyHb, which is about 24 hours in humans. In the reperfusion of ischemic rat intestine, polyHb-CAT-SOD significantly reduced the increase in oxygen radicals caused by polyHb, as measured by an increase in 3,4 dihydroxybenzoate.[14]

The author and colleagues also performed studies of global cerebral ischemia-reperfusion in a hemorrhagic shock model.[15] This was based on bleeding anesthetized rats to a hypotensive level combined with transient occlusion of both common carotid arteries. After different lengths of time, this was followed by the release of the occlusion of the carotid arteries and reinfusion using different types of oxygen-carrying fluids. The effect on the blood-brain barrier was followed by Evans

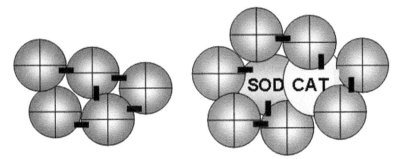

Fig.1. *Left:* PolyHb formed by nanobiotechnological assembling of Hb molecules into soluble nanodimension complex. *Right:* PolyHb-CAT-SOD formed by nanobiotechnological assembling of Hb, CAT, and SOD into soluble nanodimension complex. (*From* Chang TMS. Artificial cells: biotechnology, nanotechnology, blood substitutes, regenerative medicine, bioencapsulation. Singapore: World Scientific Publishing Co., 2007; with permission.)

blue extravasation. PolyHb-SOD-CAT, which significantly attenuated the severity of blood-brain–barrier disruption as compared with the use of saline, stroma-free Hb (SF-Hb), polyHb, or a solution of free Hb, SOD, and CAT ($P<.01$).[15,16] In the same study, brain edema was followed based on changes in brain water content. The changes in the brain water content of animals treated with polyHb-SOD-CAT were not significantly different from those of animals in the sham control group (**Figs. 2** and **3**). The increases in water content of the animals treated with saline, SF-Hb,

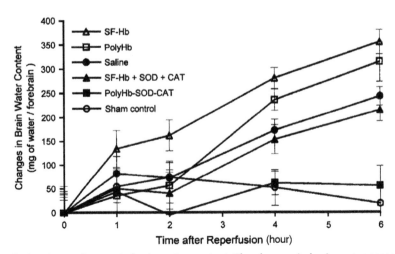

Fig. 2. Brain edema: changes in brain water content. The changes in brain water content of polyHb-SOD-CAT–treated animals are not significantly different from those of animals in the sham control group. The increases in water contents of animals treated with saline, SF-Hb, SF-Hb + SOD + CAT, and polyHb were significantly higher than those of animals in the sham control group and the polyHb-SOD-CAT group by the fourth hour and continued to increase thereafter. Statistical significance is $P<.01$. (*From* Chang TMS. Artificial cells: biotechnology, nanotechnology, blood substitutes, regenerative medicine, bioencapsulation. Singapore: World Scientific Publishing Co., 2007; with permission.)

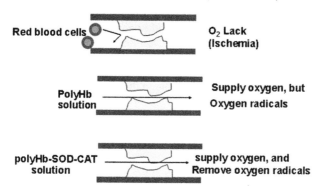

Fig. 3. In obstructive ischemia, rbc cannot pass through, but polyHb being in solution can supply oxygen but may cause ischemia-reperfusion injuries. On the other hand, polyHb-SOD-CAT can supply oxygen without causing ischemia-reperfusion injuries. (*From* Chang TMS. Artificial cells: biotechnology, nanotechnology, blood substitutes, regenerative medicine, bioencapsulation. Singapore: World Scientific Publishing Co., 2007; with permission.)

polyHb, and the solution of free Hb, SOD, and CAT were significantly higher than those of the animals in the sham control and the polyHb-SOD-CAT group by the fourth hour and increased thereafter ($P<.01$).

The attenuation in ischemia-reperfusion injuries using polyHb-SOD-CAT shows significant promise for its potential role as a protective therapeutic agent in clinical situations of ischemia and oxidative stress, such as stroke, myocardial infarction, sustained severe hemorrhagic shock, organ transplantation, and cardiopulmonary bypass.

POLYHEMOGLOBIN-FIBRINOGEN: A NOVEL OXYGEN CARRIER WITH PLATELET-LIKE PROPERTIES

In high-blood-volume loss, such as in trauma patients in hemorrhagic shock who require massive blood transfusion, large-volume RBC replacement alone does not replace platelets and coagulation factors, resulting in coagulopathy and thrombocytopenia and promoting ongoing hemorrhage. The author and colleagues therefore used nanobiotechnology to develop a blood substitute that is an oxygen carrier with platelet-like properties. This is a novel blood substitute, polyHb-fibrinogen (polyHb-Fg).[17] Briefly, polyHb-Fg was prepared as follows. A fibrinogen solution of 40 mg dissolved in 4 mL of Ringer's lactate was added to the polymerizing polyHb solution 4 hours after polymerization began. After 24 hours of polymerization, the reaction was stopped by quenching with a 2.0 M lysine solution in a molar ratio of 200:1 lysine to Hb. The solutions were then dialyzed against a Ringer's lactate solution overnight.

In Vitro Experiments

Glass tubes were prepared with 250 µL or 400 µL of blood substitute. Two-hundred-and-fifty-microliter aliquots of fresh blood were added to the 250-µL aliquots of blood substitute. One-hundred-microliter aliquots of fresh blood were added to the 400-µL aliquots of blood substitute. The timing was started when the fresh blood was added. With polyHb, the clots that formed did not adhere to the glass tubes and no clotting time could be assessed. On the other hand, all of the clots that formed using polyHb-Fg stuck to the walls of the glass tube and could be quantified with a clotting time ($P<.01$).

In Vivo Experiments

The results of in vivo experiments are shown in **Fig. 4**. polyHb displayed clotting times similar to those of polyHb-Fg for exchange transfusion of up to approximately 80%. Beyond 80% exchange, polyHb clots that formed did not always stick to the sides of the tubes and would slide freely. Beyond 93% exchange, no clots stuck for polyHb. In contrast, the clotting times for polyHb-Fg remained normal up to 98% exchange, at which point there was only a slight increase in the clotting time (see **Fig. 4**).

BIODEGRADABLE POLYMERIC NANODIMENSION ARTIFICIAL RED BLOOD CELLS

For this study, the author made use of his background in the use of the biodegradable polymers such as polylactides for artificial cells containing Hb and other biologically active material.[18] These biodegradable polymers are in routine use in surgical sutures, drug delivery, and other applications. The author is now using them to prepare nanodimension biodegradable polymer-membrane Hb with a mean diameter of between 80–200 nanometers (**Fig. 5**).[19–22] Polylactides are degraded in the body into lactic acid and then water and carbon dioxide. For a 500 mL suspension, the total lactic acid produced is 83 mEq.[5] This is far less than the normal resting-body lactic acid production (1000–1400 mEq/day). This is equivalent to 1% of the capacity of the body to breakdown lactic acid (7080 mEq/day).

In Vitro Experiments

Bovine Hb in these nanodimension artificial RBCs has the same P_{50}, Bohr, and Hill coefficients.[4–6] The content of Hb can match that of RBCs.[4–6] One can extract the whole content of RBCs and then nanoencapsulate this extract. Furthermore, additional enzymes can be added to the solution before the nanoencapsulation process. Thus, additional SOD and CAT can also be included with the Hb. The author also used his background in artificial cells containing multienzyme cofactor recycling systems[23] to help solve the problem of methemoglobin formation. In nanoRBCs, the biodegradable polymeric membranes can be made permeable to glucose and other molecules. This allows us to prepare Hb nanocapsules containing the methemoglobin reductase system in which external glucose can diffuse into the nanocapsules. Products of the reaction can diffuse out and therefore do not accumulate in the nanocapsules and inhibit the reaction. In vitro study shows that this can convert

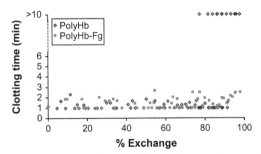

Fig. 4. Exchange transfusion using polyHb-Fg did not change the clotting time. However, exchange transfusion of polyHb of more than 80% resulted in clotting problems because there were insufficient platelets or clotting factors. (*From* Wong N, Chang TMS. Polyhemoglobin-fibrinogen a novel blood substitute with platelet-like activity for extreme hemodilution. Artif Cells Blood Substit Biotechnol, 2007; with permission.)

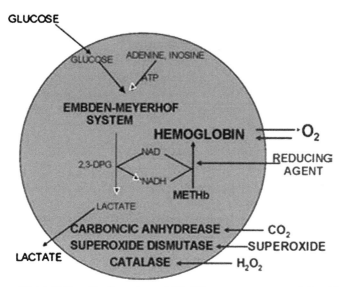

Fig. 5. Nanoartificial RBCs with diameters of 80–100 nanometers containing Hb and RBC enzymes. (*From* Chang TMS. Artificial cells: biotechnology, nanotechnology, blood substitutes, regenerative medicine, bioencapsulation. Singapore: World Scientific Publishing Co., 2007; with permission.)

methemoglobin to Hb.[19,24] Furthermore, reducing agents from the plasma can diffuse into the nanocapsules to reduce methemoglobin to oxygen-carrying Hb.[19,24]

In Vivo Experiments

Rats have been infused with one-third of the total blood volume. Most recently, the author and colleagues used a composite biodegradable polymeric membrane consisting of copolymer of polyethylene glycol (PEG) with polylactic acid (PLA).[24] After extensive research using this approach, they have now prepared nanodimension artificial RBCs that can retain their circulating Hb level at double the duration of polyHb.[24] They investigated the long-term effects of PEG-PLA nanoartificial cells containing Hb (nanoRBCs) on renal and liver function and also examined the renal, liver, and spleen histologic effects after one-third blood volume top loading in rats.[25,26] The experimental rats received one of the following infusions: nanoRBCs in Ringer lactate, Ringer lactate, SF-Hb, polyHb, or autologous rat whole blood (rat RBC). Blood samples for biochemical analysis were taken before infusion and on days 1, 7, and 21 after infusion. Rats were killed on day 21, and the kidneys, liver, and spleen were excised for histologic examination. Infusion of SF-Hb induced significant decrease in renal function, as shown by elevated levels of serum urea, creatinine, and uric acid throughout the 21 days. Histologic examination of the kidneys in the SF-Hb–infusion group revealed focal tubular necrosis and intraluminal cellular debris in the proximal tubules. In all the other groups, there were no abnormalities in renal biochemistry or histology. In conclusion, injection of nanoRBCs did not have adverse effects on renal function or renal histology. NanoRBCs, polyHb, Ringer lactate, and rat RBCs did not have any significant adverse effects on alanine aminotransferase, aspartate aminotransferase, alkaline phosphatase, creatine kinase, and amylase. On the other hand SF-Hb induced significant adverse effect on the liver, as shown by elevation in alanine aminotransferase and aspartate aminotransferase throughout the 21 days. On day 21, the rats were killed and the livers and spleens were excised for histologic examination. NanoRBCs, polyHb, Ringer's lactate, and rat RBCs did not cause any abnormalities, as seen in the microscopic histologic examination of the livers and spleens. In the SF-Hb group, the livers showed accumulation of Hb in central veins and sinusoids, and hepatic steatosis. In conclusion, injected nanoRBCs can be efficiently metabolized and removed by the reticuloendothelial system, and do not have biochemical or histologic adverse effects on the livers or the spleens.

OTHER DIRECTIONS USING NANOBIOTECHNOLOGY

The above review only includes some examples to show the use of nanobiotechnology for the preparation of blood substitutes. This principle can be extended to other systems. One example is the study conducted by the author and colleagues of another soluble nanodimension complex of polyHb-tyrosinase.[27,28] This substance has the combined function of increasing oxygen tension to sensitize melanoma to therapy and lowering systemic tyrosine to retard the growth of melanoma. Many other extensions and modifications of this general principle in nanobiotechnology are possible.[28]

SUMMARY

There is always the discussion of how safe are blood substitutes. It is reasonable to require that RBC substitutes should be able to replace allogeneic RBCs without causing more adverse effects than allogeneic RBCs. One of the safety concerns regarding RBC substitutes is related to vasoactivity. As discussed above, not all Hb-based blood substitutes have problems related to vasoactivity, and such problems are only seen in those that contain a high proportion of tetrameric Hb. The other potential problem is related to the inappropriate use of Hb-based blood substitutes in those conditions that have potential for ischemia-reperfusion injuries. For these conditions, one needs to consider use of polyHb–CAT-SOD as discussed earlier in the article.

If these precautions are followed, some of the better Hb-based blood substitutes could possibly be safer that standard allogeneic blood. After all, recent reviews show that liberal blood transfusions are associated with a 20% increase in mortality and a 56% increase in ischemic events when compared with restrictive strategies.[29,30] The transfusion of stored packed RBCs is also associated with an increase in ischemic coronary events.[29,31] In summary, although it is important for blood substitutes to be as safe as allogeneic blood, it is not reasonable to require that RBC substitutes should have no side effects whereas standard donor RBCs are associated with adverse effects including ischemic coronary events.

REFERENCES

1. Chang TMS. Semipermeable microcapsules. Science 1964;146(3643):523–5.
2. Chang TMS. Artificial cells. Monograph. Charles C Thomas, Springfield (IL), 1972. Available at: http://www.artcell.mcgill.ca. Accessed February 17, 2009.
3. Chang TMS. Stabilisation of enzymes by microencapsulation with a concentrated protein solution or by microencapsulation followed by cross-linking with glutaraldehyde. Biochem Biophys Res Commun 1971;44(6):1531–6.
4. Chang TMS. Artificial cells: biotechnology, nanotechnology, blood substitutes, regenerative medicine, bioencapsulation, cell/stem cell therapy. Singapore: World Science Publisher; 2007. p. 452.

5. Chang TMS. In: Blood substitutes: principles, methods, products and clinical trials, Vol 1. Basel, Switzerland: Karger; 1997. Available at: http://www.artcell.mcgill.ca. Accessed February 17, 2009.

6. Chang TMS. Nanobiotechnological modification of hemoglobin and enzymes from this laboratory. Biochim Biophys Acta 2008;1784:1435–40.

7. Chang TMS. Artificial cells: biotechnology, nanomedicine, regenerative medicine, blood substitutes, bioencapsulation and cell/stem cell therapy. Singapore: World Science Publisher; 2007. p. 31–61.

8. Perutz, MF. Stereochemical mechanism of oxygen transport by hemoglobin. Proc R Soc Lond B 1980;208:135.

9. Gould SA, Moore EE, Hoyt DB, et al. The life-sustaining capacity of human polymerized Hb when red cells might be unavailable. J Am Coll Surg 2002;195:445–52.

10. Pearce LB, Gawryl MS, Rentko VT, et al. HBOC-201 (Hb Glutamer-250 (Bovine), Hemopure): clinical studies. In: Winslow R, editor. Blood substitutes. San Diego: Academic Press; 2006. p. 437–50.

11. Moore EE, Moore FA, Fabian TC, et al. Human polymerized hemoglobin for the treatment of hermorrhagic shock when blood is unavailable: the USA multicenter trial. J Am Coll Surg 2009;208:1–13.

12. Yu BL, Liu ZC, Chang TMS, et al. PolyHb with different percentage of tetrameric Hb and effects on vasoactivity and electrocardiogram. Artif Cells Blood Substit Immobil Biotechnol 2006;34:159–75.

13. D'Agnillo F, Chang TMS. PolyHb-superoxide dismutase catalase as a blood substitute with antioxidant properties. Nat Biotechnol 1998;16(7):667–71.

14. Chang TMS, F. D'Agnillo, S. Razack, A second generation Hb based blood substitute with antioxidant activities. In: Blood substitutes: principles, methods, products and clinical trials, vol. 2. Chang, TMS, edition. Basel Karger Texas Landes, 1998;1009:175–85.

15. Powanda D, Chang TMS. Cross-linked polyHb-superoxide dismutase-catalase supplies oxygen without causing blood brain barrier disruption or brain edema in a rat model of transient global brain ischemia-reperfusion. Artif Cells Blood Substit Immobil Biotechnol 2002;30:25–42.

16. Chang TMS. A nanobiotechnologic therapeutic that transport oxygen and remove oxygen radicals: for stroke, hemorrhagic shock and related conditions. In: Chang TMS, editor. Artificial cells: biotechnology, nanomedicine, regenerative medicine, blood substitutes, bioencapsulation and cell/stem cell therapy. Singapore: World Science Publisher; 2007. p. 62–92.

17. Wong N, Chang TMS. Polyhemoglobin-fibrinogen: a novel blood substitute with platelet-like activity for extreme hemodilution. Artif Cells Blood Substit Immobil Biotechnol 2007;35:481–9.

18. Chang TMS. Biodegradable semipermeable microcapsules containing enzymes, hormones, vaccines, and other biologicals. J Bioeng 1976;1:25–32.

19. Chang TMS. Nanotechnology based artificial red blood cells. In: Chang TMS, editor. Artificial cells: biotechnology, nanomedicine, regenerative medicine, blood substitutes, bioencapsulation and cell/stem cell therapy. Singapore: World Science Publisher; 2007. p. 93–128.

20. Yu WP, Chang TMS. Submicron biodegradable polymer membrane Hb nanocapsules as potential blood substitutes: a preliminary report. Artif Cells Blood Substit Immobil Biotechnol 1994;22:889–94.

21. Yu WP, Chang TMS. Submicron biodegradable polymer membrane Hb nanocapsules as potential blood substitutes. Artif Cells Blood Substit Immobil Biotechnol 1996;24:169–84.

22. Chang TMS, Yu WP. Nanoencapsulation of Hb and RBC enzymes based on nano-technology and biodegradable polymer. In: Chang TMS, editor, Blood substitutes: principles, methods, products and clinical trials, Vol. 2. Basel: Karger; 1998. p. 216–31.

23. Chang TMS. Artificial cells with cofactor regenerating multienzyme systems. Methods Enzymol 1985;112:195–203.

24. Chang TMS, Powanda D, Yu WP. Ultrathin polyethylene-glycol-polylactide copolymer membrane nanocapsules containing polymerized Hb and enzymes as nano-dimension RBC substitutes. Artif Cells Blood Substit Immobil Biotechnol 2003;31:231–48.

25. Liu ZC, TMS Chang. Effects of PEG-PLA-nano artificial cells containing hemoglobin on kidney function and renal histology in rats. Artificial Cells Blood Substit Biotechnol 2008;36:421–30.

26. Liu ZC, TMS. Chang. Long-term effects on the histology and function of livers and spleens in rats after 33% toploading of PEG-PLA-nano artificial red blood cells. Artificial Cells, Blood Substitutes & Biotechnology 2008;36:513–24.

27. Yu BL, Chang TMS. In vitro and in vivo effects of polyHb–tyrosinase on murine B16F10 melanoma. Melanoma Res 2004;14:481–9.

28. Chang TMS. Enzyme artificial cells in substrate-dependent tumours and activation of prodrug. In: Chang TMS, editor. Artificial cells: biotechnology, nanomedicine, regenerative medicine, blood substitutes, bioencapsulation and cell/stem cell therapy. Singapore: World Science Publisher; 2007. p. 160–94.

29. Hill S, Carless P, Henry D, et al. Cochrane Database Syst Rev 2006;2:1–41.

30. Rao S, Harrington R, Califf R, et al. Relationship of blood transfusion and clinical outcomes in patients with acute coronary syndromes. JAMA 2005;293:673–4.

31. Rao SV, Jollis JG, Harrington RA, et al. Blood transfusion in patients with acute coronary syndrome. JAMA 2004;292:1555–62.

Stem Cells—A Source of Adult Red Blood Cells for Transfusion Purposes: Present and Future

Luc Douay, MD, PhD[a,b,c,*], Hélène Lapillonne, MD, PhD[a,b,c],
Ali G. Turhan, MD, PhD[d]

KEYWORDS

- Red blood cell • Transfusion • Enucleation • Hemoglobin
- Hematopoietic stem cells • ES cells • IPS

While the idea of universal and safe "artificial blood" is more than 50 years old, no one has come close to finding a way to replace white cells, which defend us against infections, or the platelets, which initiate blood coagulation in the event of bleeding. Thus, true artificial blood that contains white cells and all other blood components is still a long way off.

However, if the idea of artificial blood is limited to red blood cells (RBCs), the achievement of that dream is within reach. RBCs are primordial cells having essentially only one function: to transport and deliver oxygen to all the tissues of the body. A special pigment, hemoglobin, ensures this vital function. Most people who today talk about artificial blood are talking specifically about replacing this hemoglobin.

THE RED BLOOD CELL: CAN WE REPLACE SUCH A REFINED CELLULAR MODEL?

At first sight, RBCs seem uninteresting: a simple bag that has lost the vital elements, including its nucleus. In reality, it is a cell that has pushed its specialization—oxygen transport—to the point of eliminating all that is not useful.

[a] INSERM, UMR_S 893, Proliferation and differentiation of stem cells, F-75005, Paris, France
[b] UPMC Univ Paris 06, UMR_S 893, Proliferation and differentiation of stem cells, F-75005, Paris, France
[c] AP-HP, Hôpital Armand Trousseau, Service d'Hématologie biologique, 26 avenue du Dr Netter, 75012 Paris, France
[d] UPRES EA 3805, Division of Laboratory Hematology and Oncology, University of Poitiers, 2 Rue de la Milétrie, BP 577, F-86021, Poitiers, France
* Corresponding author. AP-HP, Hôpital Armand Trousseau, Service d'Hématologie biologique, 26 avenue du Dr Netter, 75012 Paris France.
E-mail address: luc.douay@trs.aphp.fr (L. Douay).

Crit Care Clin 25 (2009) 383–398
doi:10.1016/j.ccc.2008.12.008
0749-0704/08/$ – see front matter

However, this cell knows how to be unique. At its surface there exist more than 30 blood group families, which prohibit the transfusion of any indiscriminant type of RBC to any indiscriminant receiver. By liberating hemoglobin from this bag or by replacing it with a totally synthetic molecule, while still conserving its oxygen transport capacity, we would attain the objective of an "artificial blood" that could be given to any recipient.

Hemoglobin cannot simply be extracted from red blood cells and injected into the blood stream. This is because hemoglobin molecules are small and will thus, when not encapsulated, pass through the renal filter, leading to serious disorders. Thus, to use hemoglobin alone, it has to be encapsulated or modified chemically. What a paradox! Having removed the natural bag—the RBC—we must reconstruct a container that is totally artificial. One can try to envelope hemoglobin in a lipid coat or graft several hemoglobin molecules together to form a larger molecule that will not pass through the renal filter. It is likewise possible to produce recombinant hemoglobin by genetic engineering. However, such modifications may render the hemoglobin "foreign," and thus induce the synthesis of antibodies against this molecule. As an alternative, one could turn to artificial oxygen transporters, such as the perfluorocarbon molecules. However, these synthetic molecules are unstable in the blood stream. Hence, they cannot carry out their role of oxygenation for very long—24 to 48 hours at the most—and they can in no way provide long-term transfusion support for a patient who lacks RBCs.[1,2] So, after several decades of looking for a substitute for RBCs, no good alternative has been found. Nature is not so easy to replace.

Hematopoiesis: A System to be Tamed

If one cannot replace nature, why not "simply" copy her? We have sufficient knowledge of the biology of hematopoietic stem cells (HSCs)[3] to hope that we might generate human RBCs in the laboratory. One may reasonably predict that it will soon be possible to produce enough to transfuse "cultured" RBCs (cRBCs).[4]

If our objective is manufacture of human RBCs from HSCs for transfusion purposes, we are faced from the start with two challenges. The first is qualitative. In paradoxical fashion, this cell's simplicity is the result of a long route that led it to expel its nucleus. We therefore have to reproduce this natural pathway in the laboratory. The second is quantitative. An RBC concentrate transfused to a patient contains 2000 billion RBCs. Thus, it is not is not enough to produce a few cRBCs in the laboratory. We must also develop practical, economic technologies to produce vast numbers of cRBCs in a manufacturing environment.

HSCs represent 1 cell in 10,000 in the bone marrow. In close contact with the medullar microenvironment, they proliferate and differentiate according to a well-defined hierarchy to give rise to the different cell lines of the blood.[5] We know since the 1980s that HSCs are very numerous in umbilical cord blood.[6] One can also make them pass from the bone marrow to the blood by injecting specific growth factors, which facilitate their collection.[7] The medullar microenvironment is composed of different cells, which are grouped under the generic name of stromal cells. These cells secrete soluble factors, which regulate the production of HSCs and facilitate their interactions.[8–11]

This fundamental knowledge of hematopoiesis has enabled us to improve the practice of bone marrow grafting and to widen the concept to the grafting of HSCs from peripheral blood or umbilical cord blood. We have been trying for about 10 years to improve the grafting of HSC by increasing the numbers of these cells in the grafts. We speak of this as ex vivo expansion.[3] While working on this problem, we became tempted to force the cells to differentiate specifically to the RBC line, known as the erythroid line. This cell line nevertheless has an essential particularity: At the end of its maturation in the bone marrow, the erythroid cell expels its nucleus before entering the blood stream. This is the birth of the RBC, the only cell of the body to have a long life span, 120 days, despite the absence of a nucleus.

Prerequisites for Clinical Application

We can let our scientific imagination run wild for an instant and dream of ideal transfusion blood: universal RBCs produced automatically from an infinite source of HSCs. A system based on such universal RBCs would replace the present system based on blood from volunteer donors.

A so-called "blood pharming program" would aim at developing new technologies to enable the in vitro production of RBCs that are pure, readily available, and free of storage lesions. The ultimate goal of such a program would be the development of an automated cell culture and packaging system capable of generating transfusable amounts of universal donor (type O Rh−) RBCs using human stem cells as the starting material. The RBCs produced by the system would be the functional equivalent of donor-derived RBCs and induce no greater responses than those from normal donor-derived RBCs. The final result would be an automated culture system that would (1) maintain a self-renewing progenitor cell population; (2) support the differentiation, separation, and packaging of transfusable RBCs; and (3) be ready for submission to worldwide regulation agencies for all applicable device and transfusable cell product approvals.

To achieve these goals, revolutionary advances in research areas, such as those related to the control of progenitor cell expansion/differentiation and the development of automated bioreactors capable of automated cell manipulation and purification, would be necessary. Just an impossible dream? Let us analyze the obstacles that would need to be overcome.

Current Objectives to Enable Production of Red Blood Cells in the Laboratory

To reach complete terminal erythroid differentiation

To produce RBCs in the laboratory, techniques must be developed to reach complete terminal erythroid differentiation. Overcoming this obstacle means creating in vitro experimental conditions that satisfy three requirements: (1) stimulation of the proliferation of primitive HSCs, (2) induction of their exclusive commitment to the erythroid line, and (3) completion of their terminal maturation to the stage of enucleated cells.

We initially described[12] a protocol for the expansion of HSCs derived from cord blood in a well-defined medium without stroma, based on the sequential addition of growth factors. Starting from CD34+ cells, this protocol allowed the massive production (amplification up to 200,000 times) of pure erythroid precursors (up to 99%) containing fetal hemoglobin. Contrary to what happens under these ex vivo conditions in the presence of growth factors alone, such progenitors/precursors are capable of continuing to proliferate in vivo and of differentiating within 4 days to the terminal stage of enucleated cells producing adult hemoglobin when are injected into NOD/SCID (nonobese diabetic–severe combined immunodeficiency) mice, they are capable of continuing to proliferate in vivo and of differentiating within 4 days to the terminal stage of enucleated cells producing adult hemoglobin. This points to a major role of the microenvironment in terminal erythroid differentiation.

On the basis of these data, we subsequently modified our protocol to obtain the expansion and differentiation of CD34+ cells derived from blood, bone marrow, or cord blood in three steps:[13] (1) in a liquid medium and in the presence of stem cell factor, interleukin-3, and erythropoietin; (2) in the presence of erythropoietin alone (based on a model reconstitution of the microenvironment [murine stromal cell line

MS5]); and (3) in the presence of the stromal cells alone, without any growth factors. This cell culture system in a well-defined medium without serum reproduces ex vivo the microenvironment existing in vivo[14] (**Fig. 1**).

Using this protocol, we obtain after 15 days a plateau of the mean amplification of CD34+ cells of 20,000-fold for cells from bone marrow or peripheral blood, 30,000-fold for cells obtained by leukapheresis after mobilization with granulocyte-colony stimulating factor, and 200,000-fold for cells derived from cord blood. A total commitment to the erythroid lineage is morphologically evident after 8 days. Differentiation of the reticulocytes into mature RBCs continues from day 15 to day 18, as shown by the further disappearance of nuclei, progressive loss of transferrin receptor CD71 expression, and staining with laser dye styryl (LDS). At this stage, 90% to 100% of the cells are enucleated. These erythrocytes display characteristics close to those of native RBCs in terms of mean corpuscular volume, mean corpuscular hemoglobin, and mean corpuscular hemoglobin concentration (**Fig. 2A**).

To assess the functionality of "cultured" red blood cells

Before artificial blood can be used, the reticulocytes and cRBCs generated ex vivo have to be shown to be the functional equivalent of donor-derived RBCs.

The reticulocytes have glucose-6-phosphate dehydrogenase and pyruvate kinase levels in keeping with the properties of a young homogenous RBC population. This indicates that they are capable of reducing glutathione and maintaining adenosine triphosphate levels and therefore have a normal level of 2,3-diphosphoglycerate.

The deformability of these reticulocytes and red blood cells, as evaluated by ektacytometry, is comparable to that of native erythrocytes.[15]

The functionality of the hemoglobin present in cRBCs is assessed by ligand-binding kinetics after flash photolysis. The bimolecular kinetics after photodissociation of carbon monoxide provide a sensitive test of hemoglobin function. On varying the energy of the photolysis pulse, two phases are observed. These phases correspond to the two hemoglobin conformations (relaxed [R] and tense [T] states). The kinetics are thus biphasic, reflecting the two allosteric forms.

Like native hemoglobin, cRBC hemoglobin is able to fix and release oxygen. Oxygen equilibrium measurements confirm the observed affinity and cooperativity. The $\log(P_{50})$ value is 1.2 for cRBC hemoglobin as compared with 1.3 for control RBC

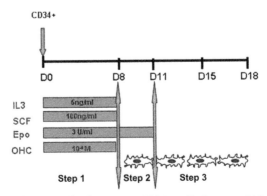

Fig. 1. Amplification of erythroid cells. Human CD34+ cells from cord blood, bone marrow, or peripheral blood are cultured in a liquid medium on a layer of stromal cells of murine origin (MS5) according to a three-phase protocol. D, day; Epo, erythropoietin; IL3, interleukin-3; OHC, hydroxycortisone; SCF, stem cell factor.

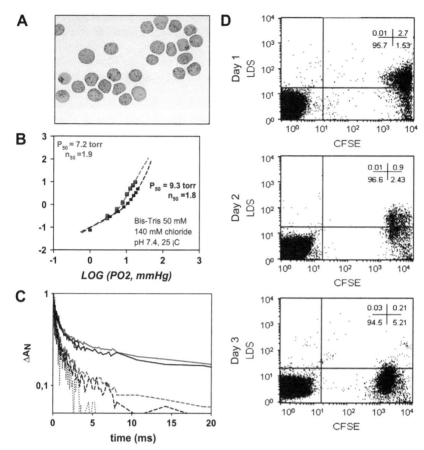

Fig. 2. Functional analysis of cRBCs. (*A*) Cells at a reticulocyte stage on day 15 of culture after May-Grünwald-Giemsa staining. (*B*) Oxygen dissociation curve at 25°C Hill plot of deoxygenation and reoxygenation of cRBCs (*red*) and normal control RBCs (*blue*). The two curves are nearly identical. Bis-Tris, 2-hydroxyethyl-hydroxymethyl; PO2; n_{50}, Hill coefficient; torr, mm Hg (*C*) Carbon monoxide rebinding after flash photolysis of hemoglobin from cRBCs (*red curves with circles*) and hemoglobin from control native RBCs (*blue curves*). The two samples show similar binding properties, including the allosteric transition. By varying the energy of the photolysis pulse, one can vary the total fraction of dissociated hemoglobin and thereby probe in detail the various partially bound populations. At high photolysis levels, more singly bound tetramers are produced, which switch to the deoxy conformation (T-state) and rebind ligands more slowly. At intermediate levels one can analyze in detail the partially bound populations. At low photolysis levels, one can better probe the doubly bound tetramers, a form difficult to study by equilibrium techniques. At sufficiently low levels, the main photoproducts are triply bound tetramers, which rebind ligands rapidly (R-state). (*D*) Flow cytometric analysis of CFSE-labeled cRBCs in the NOD SCID mouse model. (*a*) Kinetics of the expression of CFSE/LDS markers in cells from peripheral blood of the mice. (*Horizontal axis*) CFSE detection. (*Vertical axis*) LDS detection. Quadrant statistics are shown on each dot plot. (*b*) On day 3, the cells were colabeled with a phycoerythin-conjugated anti-RhD antibody (*solid histogram*) or its control isotype (*open histogram*). Results are expressed in terms of the percentage of RhD+ cells among CFSE+ cells.

hemoglobin and the Hill coefficients are identical (N_{50} of 2.28 versus 2.29). The kinetic and equilibrium data therefore indicate ligand-binding properties in very close agreement with control values. Methemoglobin is not detected, which shows that cRBCs are enzymatically capable of reversing hemoglobin oxidation (**Fig. 2** B, C).

Concerning the in vivo fate of cRBCs, after intraperitoneal infusion into NOD SCID mice, carboxyfluorescein diacetate succinimidyl ester (CFSE)–labeled cRBCs and reticulocytes obtained by apheresis persist in the circulation to the same extent as CFSE-labeled native RBCs: CFSE+ cells are detected for 3 days in both groups of transfused animals. In vivo, the transfused reticulocytes fully mature into RBCs as shown by the appearance of CFSE+/LDS− cells. Over 90% of the CFSE+ cells are mature RBCs by day 3 (**Fig. 2**D). Work is now in progress to demonstrate that cRBCs have a normal lifespan of close to 120 days in vivo in humans.

At this stage of development of the model, it has thus been established that it is possible to produce functional human cRBCs by culturing hematopoietic stem cells.

To produce large quantities of "cultured" red blood cells in vitro

For cRBCs to be practical, they must be produced in concentrations comparable to that of a standard red cell concentrate transfused to a patient (ie, 2000 billion).

Interestingly, the total cell expansion obtained during the first step of our protocol in the presence of growth factors alone is directly related to the duration of culture. When this is prolonged for 3 additional days, the level of expansion increases dramatically to reach 1×10^7-fold for cord blood or peripheral blood or 2×10^5-fold for bone marrow products, with preservation of the terminal differentiation after steps 2 and 3 (70% to 91% enucleated cells).

Considering on the one hand the levels of cell amplification obtained (2×10^5- to 1×10^7-fold for apheresis and cord blood with 90% to 100% maturation) and, on the other hand, a mean quantity of 2 to 8×10^6 CD34+ cells/kg in an apheresis donation or 2 to 5×10^6 CD34+ cells in a cord blood unit, this procedure can theoretically produce the equivalent of 5 to 10 RBC concentrates.

To design the conditions for industrial development

An automated culture and packaging system to supply RBCs must be able to produce cRBCs on a large scale and these cRBCs must be functionally equivalent to fresh donor cells, especially with regard to their oxygen-carrying capacity and morphology.

To develop such a system using various sources of progenitor cells, several significant technical challenges in the fields of cell biology and bioreactor performance and design have to be overcome. While it has been shown that mature, functional cRBCs can be derived from a number of different progenitor cell types, including those obtained from bone marrow, cord blood, and apheresis blood, large-scale production of transfusable RBCs has not yet been achieved regardless of the progenitor cell source.

An automated cell culture system capable of maintaining a self-renewing progenitor population, providing an environment for efficient differentiation along the erythroid pathway, and allowing sorting/purification and packaging of the end product RBCs in a manner directly suitable for transfusion does not yet exist. It is envisioned that an automated culture/packaging system must operate with minimal user intervention. To achieve these aims, revolutionary advances in research areas, such as the control of progenitor cell expansion/differentiation and the development of bioreactors capable of automated cell manipulation and purification, will be necessary. This is challenging, but not impossible!

To generate a universal red blood cell population
This culture system offers a new approach to the search for "universal" cRBCs (ie, RBCs lacking membrane expression of the two principal blood group systems, ABO and Rhesus D [RhD]).

While technologies for manipulation and removal of blood group antigen presentation are emerging, perhaps the simplest method could be to use exclusively materials derived from type O Rh− donors (peripheral blood or cord blood).

The concept of cRBCs opens the way to another promising approach: Rather than trying to eliminate the surface antigens once they have formed, prevent the synthesis of those antigens before the cells reach maturity. The blood group antigens ABO and Rh, which are not expressed on HSCs, are already present on erythroblast precursors. Two possible techniques can be imagined for preventing synthesis of antigens.

The first is the inhibition of gene expression in CD34+ human HSCs through the use of interfering RNA. This technique enables posttranscription inhibition of a gene in a sequence-specific manner by employing double-stranded RNA to provoke degradation of the homologous mRNA. Such inhibition of the expression of genes has been partially achieved using antisense oligonucleotides or ribozymes, but the approach is limited by the instability of the molecules introduced. The second possibility is the biochemical intracellular inhibition of the glycosyltransferases specific for the antigens A and B.

Whatever the mechanism, this inhibition has to be initiated at the stage of CD34+ HSCs and continued to that of cRBCs. The methods of this approach can in fact avoid the side effects inherent to the procedures of antigen stripping[16] or masking[17] currently being tested.

Tomorrow's Perspectives: to Create New Sources of Hematopoietic Stem Cells

The use of human stem cells for several potential therapeutic applications implies that they can be differentiated in vitro into cells entirely similar to their natural counterpart. Human embryonic stem cells (huESCs) and the recently described induced pluripotent stem cells (iPSCs) represent a promising source of progenitors for specific tissue cell production. However, the difficulties of using this source have not yet been completely solved and no one can be sure that a few weeks of culture in vitro will be able to reproduce the long natural in vivo maturation process. In this context, erythropoiesis is an instructive model. Thus, while we have demonstrated that it is possible to recapitulate complete terminal erythropoiesis in vitro starting from adult or cord blood HSCs, no one has succeeded in generating fully mature RBCs (ie, enucleated and containing adult hemoglobin) from primitive stem cells. We will review here these exciting possibilities.

FETAL AND EMBRYONIC STEM CELL SOURCES
Undifferentiated Human Embryonic Stem Cells

First isolated in 1998, huESCs are derived from the inner cell mass of the blastocyte stage of the human embryo.[18] After immunosurgical isolation and under appropriate culture conditions, the inner cell mass cells give rise to huESC lines. Human ESCs are undifferentiated, pluripotent cells that can be maintained indefinitely in culture on mouse embryonic feeder cells in the presence of basic fibroblast growth factor. These cells express (1) specific cell surface markers, such as stage-specific embryonic antigen (SSEA)-3, SSEA-4, tumor rejection antigen (Tra)-1-60, and Tra-1-81; and (2) specific genes, such as *Oct3/4*, *Nanog*, and *Sox2*, which are involved in the maintenance of their pluripotency capacity. ESCs maintain a normal karyotype and high telomerase activity and are distinguished by their capacity to differentiate in vitro and in vivo into tissues derived from all three embryonic germ-cell layers (ectoderm, endoderm, and mesoderm), the mesoderm layer giving rise to hematopoietic cells. In 2006, more than 400 cell lines were registered around the world. Human ESCs provide a unique alternative to the early embryo for study of the more primitive stages of development and an unlimited starting population of cells for investigation of human hematopoietic commitment and, more specifically, terminal erythropoiesis for transfusion and transplantation purposes.[19,20]

Hematopoietic Development

During mammalian embryogenesis, the hematopoietic system is established in two waves termed *primitive* and *definitive*.[21] Primitive hematopoiesis is initiated in the extraembryonic yolk sac within blood islands comprised of primitive erythroblasts, mature macrophages, and mast cells surrounded by endothelial cells. Primitive erythropoiesis is transient from 14 to 19 days postconception until the ninth week of embryonic development and generates megaloblastic nucleated erythroid cells producing embryonic globins. Definitive hematopoiesis is initiated in the aorto-gonado-mesonephros (AGM) region of the embryo. This region is the source of the first HSCs capable of reconstituting adult host hematopoiesis. During the sixth week of gestation, the definitive site of hematopoiesis shifts to the fetal liver and then to the bone marrow, where all adult-type lineages are produced. Definitive erythropoiesis produces normocytic enucleated erythrocytes that synthesize fetal globins followed by adult globins. Interestingly, there is compelling evidence that both yolk sac– and AGM-derived HSCs are the direct progeny of a bipotential hemato/endothelial cell called the hemangioblast.

Hematopoietic Differentiation from Human Embryonic Stem Cells

Undifferentiated huESCs already express some cell surface markers and genes known to be characteristic of HSCs: (1) the CD117 (c-kit), CD133 (AC133) and CD90 (thy-1) surface markers and (2) the LMO2, AML1, and c-MYB genes. These cells also express the KDR/flk1 (kinase insert domain protein receptor/fetal liver kinase–1) and FLT-1 (Fms-related tyrosine kinase–1) genes more specific to the endothelial pathway.

After removal from the feeder cells and withdrawal of basic fibroblast growth factor, two main experimental techniques are used to initiate huESC differentiation: formation of embryoid bodies or coculture on supportive stromal cell layers (**Fig. 3**).

Hematopoietic differentiation by embryoid body formation

Suspension cultures of huESC form embryoid bodies, which are three-dimensional aggregates of colonies of differentiated cells, including mesoderm-derived cells. A combination of five cytokines (stem cell factor, FLT3-L [Fms-related tyrosine kinase 3 ligand], interleukin-3, interleukin-6, and granulocyte-colony stimulating factor) and bone morphogenetic protein-4, a ventral mesoderm inducer, strongly promotes hematopoietic differentiation,[22–24] while addition of vascular endothelial growth factor (VEGF-A$_{165}$) promotes erythropoiesis.[25] The hematopoietic and erythroid commitments are assessed by analyzing cell surface antigens by flow cytometry (CD34, CD38, CD45, CD31, CD41a, and CD235a), gene expression by real-time reverse transcription polymerase chain reaction (GATA-1, GATA-2, SCL/TAL-1 [stem cell leukemia/T-cell acute leukemia–1], EKLF [erythroid Krüppel-like factor], PU-1, and globins), and formation of clonogenic progenitors by colony-forming unit (CFU) assay. Gordon Keller's group has shown that 72 to 96 hours of embryoid body differentiation

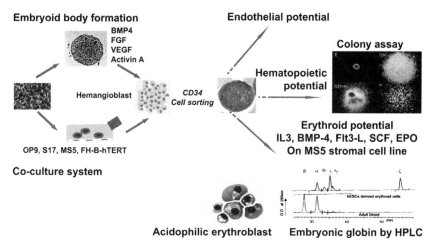

Embryoid body formation

BMP4
FGF
VEGF
Activin A

Hemangioblast

CD34
Cell sorting

OP9, S17, MS5, FH-B-hTERT

Co-culture system

Endothelial potential

Colony assay

Hematopoietic
potential

Erythroid potential
IL3, BMP-4, Flt3-L, SCF, EPO
On MS5 stromal cell line

Acidophilic erythroblast   **Embryonic globin by HPLC**

Fig. 3. Hematopoietic differentiation from huESC. See text. BMP4, bone morphogenetic protein-4; FGF, fibroblast-derived growth factor; VEGF, vascular endothelial growth factor; IL3, interleukin-3; Flt3-L, fetal liver tyrosine kinase 3 ligand; SCF, stem cell factor; EPO, erythropoietin; HPLC, high-performance liquid chromatography.

produces blast cell colonies co-expressing KDR and CD117. These human blast colonies have hematopoietic and endothelial potential: The adherent cells generate colonies expressing different vascular genes, including *KDR* and *CD31*, while the non-adherent population expresses embryonic globin genes and GATA-1.[26] Bhatia's and Civin's groups[22,25,27] found that during embryoid body differentiation CD34+ cells appeared as early as day 5, peaked by day 12 to day 15, and represented up to 10% of the total population. All types of colonies are produced by differentiated huESCs, including colony forming units-erythroid (CFU-E), CFU–granulocyte macrophage (CFU-GM), CFU–erythrocyte, monocyte/macrophage, megakaryocyte (CFU-GEMM), burst-forming unit–erythroid, and CFU-megakaryocyte. While 7 to 12 days of embryoid body differentiation seems to give rise to adherent and nonadherent cells with more primitive hematopoiesis expressing embryonic and fetal globin genes, 12 to 20 days of embryoid body differentiation results in more definitive hematopoiesis with little β-globin gene expression. The emergence of primitive erythropoiesis coincides with an increase in the expression of *SCL/TAL-1*, *GATA-1*, *GATA-2*, *EKLF*, *C-MYB*, and *PU-1*. The main advantage of embryoid body differentiation is that it mimics human yolk sac development and the waves of hematopoietic commitment.[28]

Hematopoietic differentiation in coculture systems
The second approach used to promote hematopoiesis is to coculture undifferentiated huESCs on supportive stromal cell lines, such as S17 cells (from mouse bone marrow), C116 cells (from embryonic mouse yolk sacs), MS5 cells (from mouse bone marrow), OP9 cells (macrophage colony stimulating factor–deficient cells from mouse bone marrow), or FH-B-hTERT cells (from human fetal liver);[29–32]
Slukvin's group[30] found that differentiation of huESCs in coculture with OP9 cells produced 5- to 10-fold more hematopoietic progenitors and stem cells as compared with coculture with S17, C116, or MS5 cell lines. These investigators were able to obtain up to 20% CD34+ cells. In OP9 cocultures, CD34+ cells first appeared on day 3, followed by CD31 cells on day 4, CD41a and CD43 cells on day 5, and CD45 cells on day 8. Concomitantly, CFU-E colonies emerged first, followed by

CFU–GEMM, CFU–GM, and CFU-granulocyte colonies, while GATA-1 and GATA-2 gene expression was detected on day 3 followed by *SCL/TAL-1* expression on day 4. CD43 (leukosialin)[33] was also identified as an interesting marker (1) to detect clonogenic progenitors before expression of CD45, (2) to follow hematopoietic differentiation, and (3) to separate the CD34+ hematopoietic population from CD34+CD43−CD31+KDR+ endothelial and CD34+CD43−CD31−KDR− mesenchymal cells. Two major populations of hematopoietic progenitors were present: (1) CD43+CD235a+CD41a+CD45− cells with restricted erythroid and megakaryocytic potential and (2) CD43+CD45+/−Lin− multilineage progenitors, where CD45−Lin− cells displayed lymphomyeloid and CD45+Lin− cells displayed progressive myeloid commitment.

Erythroid differentiation from human embryonic stem cells

Over the last few years, Bouhassira's group[32,34] has established a protocol to promote erythropoietic differentiation. Undifferentiated huESC cocultured with FH-B-hTERT cells can generate 1.9% to 9% CD34+ cells. In a four-step liquid culture protocol, the CD34-sorted cells can then be differentiated into a pure erythroid population. Interestingly, increasing the duration of coculture on FH-B-hTERT cells from 14 days to 21 or 35 days led to (1) a respective 32-, 129-, and 846-fold increase in the absolute number of erythroid cells; (2) differentiation of megaloblastic nucleated erythroblasts to give 6.5% macroblastic enucleated RBCs after 35 days of coculture; and (3) an increase in α versus ζ and γ versus ϵ globin chains as detected by high-performance liquid chromatography.[35] The investigators did not show results for tetrameric hemoglobin but concluded that there must be partial replacement of hemoglobin Gower I ($\zeta 2\epsilon 2$) by Gower II ($\alpha 2\epsilon 2$) before hemoglobin F ($\alpha 2\gamma 2$). No β-globin protein was detectable by high-performance liquid chromatography and only traces of the mRNA by real-time polymerase chain reaction. This in vitro protocol mimics the major hemoglobin switches observed between weeks 4 and 9 during human embryonic development. Similar percentages of enucleated RBCs were obtained using differentiated huESC or fetal liver cells.

Human Fetal Liver Cells and Mouse Embryonic Stem Cells

On the basis of these observations, we and others have investigated the capacity of an intermediate ontogenic source, human fetal liver, to expand and differentiate into erythroid lineage cells. We cocultured CD34+ cells derived from 13-week fetal liver for up to 18 days on an in vitro reconstitution of the bone marrow microenvironment in a medium containing cytokines. While a dramatic cell expansion was observed with complete induction of erythropoiesis, less than 15% of the total cells achieved terminal differentiation into mature RBCs producing fetal hemoglobin. Interestingly, the hemoglobin content and rate of enucleation seemed to correlate with the developmental age of the CD34+ cells (personal data, 2008).

Using mouse embryonic stem cells, Carotta and colleagues[36] have developed a three-step protocol to generate mass cultures of pure, immature erythroid progenitors capable of differentiating into mature enucleated erythrocytes. Starting from 20,000 mouse ESCs and combining embryoid body differentiation with erythroid culture conditions, these investigators were able to produce more than 10^{11} erythroid progenitors within 10 weeks. After 14 days' culture, the erythroid cells exclusively expressed the adult β-globin gene.

Many studies are being performed with huESCs. However, although hematopoietic induction of huESCs is quite routinely attained by several teams, none has yet succeeded in obtaining mature cells, such as RBCs. To reach that holy grail, a lot of work needs to be done and a number of different problems must be solved: (1) the proliferative potential must be increased beyond the current expansion limit of 2000- to 10,000-fold; (2) techniques must be developed to bring about terminal erythroid maturation, which so far has not been achieved because the cells do not enucleate and resemble the primitive erythroid cells present in the yolk sac of early embryos; and (3) ways must be found to address the problem of content in erythroid cells, which now have a major embryonic/fetal globin content, expressing less than 2% adult β-globin mRNA.

ADULT PLURIPOTENT STEM CELL SOURCES
Multipotent Adult Progenitor Cells

During the last few years, several studies have clearly demonstrated the possibility of isolating primitive multipotent stem cells from adult human tissues. The initial work of Verfaillie and colleagues[37] showed that it is possible to isolate a stem cell from the adult tissues of mice and humans using techniques of negative selection (depletion of cells expressing differentiation antigens) and extensive low-density culture in the presence of low concentrations of serum (2.5% fetal calf serum) and a combination of endothelial growth factor and platelet-derived growth factor. The cells that can be obtained by this procedure, designated as multipotent adult progenitor cells (MAPCs), exhibit very few differentiation markers but express Oct4, the major transcription factor identified in embryonic stem cells. Most importantly, these cells have a high proliferative potential (up to 120 divisions), which could be of major interest for the production of mature hematopoietic cells. It was difficult to elicit the hematopoietic potential of MAPCs until the discovery that only MAPCs with high Oct4 expression were able to generate hematopoietic cells in vitro and in vivo in mice. The difficulty of obtaining MAPC reproducibly from different adult tissues has discouraged several laboratories, but other stem cell populations with characteristics similar to those of MAPCs have recently been isolated from adult tissues.

Unrestricted Somatic Stem Cells

Kogler and colleagues[38] have shown that it is possible to isolate from cord blood, after 2 to 4 weeks in culture, a cell population termed *unrestricted somatic stem cells* (USSCs). These cells display characteristics of pluripotent stem cells and their culture conditions appear to be much more suitable for potential clinical use. Thus, at the end of the culture procedure, adherent colonies were detected in the dishes with a frequency of four colonies per cord blood sample and these cells could further undergo major expansion, up to a theoretical number of 10^{15} cells.[38] These cells could be induced to differentiate into mesodermal, neuroectodermal, and endodermal layers, with evidence of in vitro generation of neural cells, osteoblasts, cardiomyocytes, and liver cells. After intrauterine injection in a sheep model, they could generate human hematopoietic cells detectable in vivo for several months,[38] suggesting that they were capable of self-renewal and differentiation in vivo. Given that cord blood is a stem cell source already in clinical use, USSCs can be of interest for cRBC generation. However, specific culture conditions must be in place before one can exploit such a possibility. First, a sufficient number of cord blood samples must be available to supply USSCs. The initial work suggested that only 30% of cord blood samples contain such cell populations (94 among 233 tested). This problem could easily be solved if a large banking effort from the existing cord blood banks was made for USSC generation. The second condition is proof that HSCs can be generated from USSCs, which is a critical step similar to the challenge we are facing when dealing with huESCs. The culture conditions for these cells to differentiate not only into meso-dermal cells but also into HSCs will have to be established before attempting to produce cRBCs from their progeny. This problem is likely to be analogous to that of establishing the culture conditions to elicit HSC potential from huESCs.

Diverse Potential Sources of Multipotent Stem Cells

Several teams have described other types of "multipotent" stem cells obtained from bone marrow, skin, fat tissue, and, more recently, human amniocytic fluid.[39] This last source is interesting because it is readily accessible and clinical banking procedures could easily be set up. The stem cells, called *amniotic fluid–derived stem cells* (AFSCs), can be obtained by selection of c-kit+ cells from cultures in minimum essential medium in the presence of 15% fetal calf serum. Clonal, adherent c-kit+ cells can thus be identified and amplified (up to 250 population doublings). AFSCs exhibit long telomeres and a normal karyotype and appear to be nontumorigenic in immunodeficient mice.[39] These cells are CD34−, CD45−, and CD133− and express markers characteristic of ESCs, including Oct4 and Tra-1-81. In the original work, they were found to be capable of generating muscle and hepatocytelike cells,[39] but their hematopoietic potential and especially their ability to generate RBCs remains to be determined.

Patient-Specific Stem Cells

One potential clinical problem facing all the multipotent stem cell types described (although less challenging than that of HSC generation) is the potential immunogenicity of these cells. This question, which is also valid for huESC lines, has led some investigators to test the possibility of generating patient-specific stem cells. One approach, which has been studied extensively in mice, is the production of cells like ESCs by therapeutic cloning.[40] This technique allows the reprogramming of an adult somatic cell nucleus in the microenvironment, provided by an oocyte from which the nucleus has been removed by micromanipulation. After nuclear transfer, the oocyte undergoes symmetric divisions and a blastocystlike structure is obtained in vitro. The internal cell mass of this structure can then be used to generate an ESC line that in turn produces differentiated adult tissues in vitro, expressing the histocompatibility antigens of the nucleus donor. These cells suggest exciting possibilities for cell and gene therapy,[40] but also potentially for the generation of RBCs if the hurdles of hematopoietic induction and final RBC maturation can be cleared. The major practical difficulties of this approach are the problem of the availability of oocyte donors and the ethical concern. A large-scale clinical application for RBC production after nuclear transfer currently appears to be difficult, unless the present work with huESCs achieves a major breakthrough leading to a reproducible and clinically applicable method of inducing the HSC commitment of mesoderm and robust methods of RBC generation.

The Latest Revolution: Induced Pluripotent Stem Cells

In the search for novel sources of pluripotent stem cells, the recent discovery of the possibility of inducing a pluripotent stem cell state in an adult cell has profoundly affected the field of stem cell research. The pioneering work in this domain may be credited to Yamanaka's group,[41] which performed an in-depth screening of all the pluripotency genes sufficient and necessary for the induction of an ESC-like state in adult cells. The group identified four pluripotency factors and showed that enforced expression of these four pluripotency genes (*Oct4*, *Klf4*, *Sox2*, and *c-myc*) was sufficient to generate a pluripotent "stem cell state" in a murine embryonic or adult fibroblast, which acquired an embryonic stem cell phenotype.[41] The embryonic cell line obtained by this procedure contributed to all adult tissues after injection into blastocysts, generated teratomas in immunodeficient mice, and expressed markers similar to those of genuine murine ESCs.[41] During the initial iPSC isolation, Yamanaka's group used a mouse strain in which the *Fbx15* locus, one of the targets of *Oct4*, was placed before the G418R gene by a procedure of homologous recombination. Cells expressing Oct4 were thus identified by the appearance of G418-resistant cells and also by their characteristic ESC-like morphology. The ESC colony taken from the culture was able to grow under ESC conditions on mouse embryonic feeder layers in the presence of leukemia inhibitory factor.[41] An important step in confirming the embryonic nature of the cells was the demonstration of the ability of iPSCs to acquire germline transmission potential.[42,43] However, myc-gene overexpression induced tumors in mice [42] and more recent data have shown that transfer of three genes (*Oct4*, *Klf4*, and *Sox2*) was sufficient to induce a pluripotent state.

The prospects for iPSC technology have been further improved by the demonstration of the feasibility of this approach in human cells.[44,45] These recent data indicate that expression of the four "Yamanaka genes" could be sufficient for iPSC generation, but that primary human fibroblasts and mesenchymal stem cells appear to be difficult to reprogram unless they express hTERT and the SV40 large T antigen.[44,45] Strikingly, the cells that reverted to an "ESC-like" phenotype could be identified in these cultures by their morphology and expanded thereafter under huESC conditions.[44,45] The iPSCs obtained from human mesenchymal stem cells have further been shown to be able to generate hematopoietic cells.[44]

While iPSC technology has sparked enthusiasm, many difficulties remain with regard to the reproducible generation of iPSC lines from adult tissues and the challenge of producing HSCs and RBCs for transfusion purposes from these cells. The major advantage of iPSC technology is the autologous nature of the cells, which circumvents the problem of immunogenicity. Several questions remain concerning the amplification potential of these cells, their genetic stability, and their absence of tumorigenicity. The concerns raised by use of insertional mutagenesis could be eliminated if the programming could be performed by means of passively diffusing

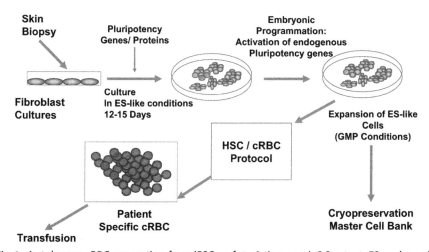

Fig. 4. Autologous cRBC generation from iPSCs: a futuristic scenario? See text. ES, embryonic stem; GMP, good manufacturing practices.

proteins or small molecules involved in the signaling pathways of the pluripotency genes.

A possible futuristic scenario for cRBC generation is illustrated in **Fig. 3**. If this scenario becomes a reality within this century, a simple skin biopsy could be used to generate a bank of master iPSCs from an adult with aplastic anemia or myeloid leukemia. These cells could then be amplified and induced to differentiate into mesodermal cells and subsequently into HSCs for cRBC production (**Fig. 4**). One important step toward this futuristic goal was recently achieved in a mouse model of sickle cell anemia by transplantation of hematopoietic cells generated by iPSC methods after correction of the sickle cell abnormality by homologous recombination.[46]

SUMMARY

Though the notion of artificial blood has been talked about a long time, we are still waiting for authentic blood substitutes. Perhaps this is a sign that, at least in the case of blood cells, it is not easy to replace nature. However, as the concept of the cRBC shows, it is nevertheless possible to imitate nature. Now remains the task of designing the industrial conditions for the development of this approach and to demonstrate the clinical and economic value of this new blood product with simple characteristics: a concentrate of homogeneous RBCs that have a long life span and a selected phenotype; that are free of platelets, leukocytes, and plasma; and that offer improved storage characteristics over conventional RBCs; and that are reliably and readily available. It further remains to be determined whether autologous stem cell sources or huESC-derived cells will be the best candidates for future development. The road to the production line will be long, 5 to 10 years perhaps. In other words, tomorrow!

REFERENCES

1. Creteur J, Sibbald W, Vincent J, et al. Hemoglobin solutions—not just red blood cell substitutes. Crit Care Med 2000;28:3025–34.
2. Spahn DR, Waschke KF, Standl T, et al. Use of perflubron emulsion to decrease allogenic blood transfusion in high-blood-loss non-cardiac surgery: results of a European phase 3 study. Anesthesiology 2002;97:1338–49.
3. Douay L. Experimental culture conditions are critical for ex vivo expansion of hematopoietic cells. J Hematother Stem Cell Res 2001;21:341–6 [Review].
4. Douay L, Andreu G. Ex vivo production of human red blood cells from hematopoietic stem cells: What is the future in transfusion? Transfus Med Rev 2007;2: 91–100.
5. Ogawa M. Differentiation and proliferation of hematopoietic stem cells. Blood 1993;81:2844–53.
6. Lu L, Xiaa M, Shen PN, et al. Enrichment, characterization, and responsiveness of single primitive CD34 human umbilical cord blood hematopoietic progenitors with high proliferative and replating potential. Blood 1993;81(1):41–8.
7. Firat H, Douay L. Ex vivo expansion of mobilized peripheral blood stem cells. Baillieres Best Pract Res Clin Haematol 1999;12(1–2):99–115.
8. Friedenstein AJ, et al. Precursors for fibroblasts in different populations of hematopoietic cells as detected by the in vitro colony assay method. Exp Hematol 1974;2:83–92.
9. Koller MR, Oxender M, Jensen TC, et al. Direct contact between CD34+lin- cells and stroma induces a soluble activity that specifically increases primitive hematopoietic cell production. Exp Hematol 1999;27:734–41.

10. Lemischka IR. Microenvironmental regulation of hematopoietic stem cells. Stem Cells 1997;1(15 Suppl):63–8.
11. Verfaillie CM. Soluble factor(s) produced by human bone marrow stroma increase cytokine-induced proliferation and maturation of primitive hematopoietic progenitors while preventing their terminal differentiation. Blood 1993;82:2045–53.
12. Neildez-Nguyen TMA, Wajcman H, Marden MC, et al. Human erythroid cells produced ex vivo at large scale differentiate into red blood cells in vivo. Nat Biotechnol 2002;5:467–72.
13. Giarratana MC, Kobari L, Lapillonne H, et al. Ex vivo generation of fully mature human red blood cells from hematopoietic stem cells. Nat Biotechnol 2005;23(1):69–74.
14. Lichtman MA. The ultrastructure of the hemopoietic environment of the marrow: a review. Exp Hematol 1981;9:391–410.
15. Cynober T, Mohandas N, Tchernia G, et al. Red cell abnormalities in hereditary spherocytosis: relevance to diagnosis and understanding of the variable expression of clinical severity. J Lab Clin Med 1996;128:259–69.
16. Kruskall MS, AuBuchon JP, Anthony KY, et al. Transfusion to blood group A and O patients of group B RBCs that have been enzymatically converted to group O. Transfusion 2000;40(11):1290–8.
17. Nacharaju P, Boctor F, Manjoula B, et al. Surface decoration of red blood cells with maleimidophenyl-polyethylene glycol facilitated by thiolation with iminothiolane: an approach to mask A, B, and D antigens to generate universal red blood cells. Transfusion 2005;45:374–83.
18. Thomson JA, Itskovitz-Eldor J, Shapiro SS, et al. Embryonic stem cell lines derived from human blastocysts. Science 1998;282(5391):1145–7.
19. Keller G. Embryonic stem cell differentiation: emergence of a new era in biology and medicine. Genes Dev 2005;19(10):1129–55.
20. Olsen AL, Stachura DL, Weiss MJ, et al. Designer blood: creating hematopoietic lineages from embryonic stem cells. Blood 2006;107(4):1265–75.
21. Kingsley PD, Malik J, Fantauzzo KA, et al. Yolk sac–derived primitive erythroblasts enucleate during mammalian embryogenesis. Blood 2004;104(1):19–25.
22. Chadwick K, Wang L, Li L, et al. Cytokines and BMP-4 promote hematopoietic differentiation of human embryonic stem cells. Blood 2003;102(3):906–15.
23. Woll PS, Martin CH, Miller JS, et al. Human embryonic stem cell–derived NK cells acquire functional receptors and cytolytic activity. J Immunol 2005;175(8):5095–103.
24. Galic Z, Kitchen SG, Kacena A, et al. T lineage differentiation from human embryonic stem cells. Proc Natl Acad Sci U S A 2006;103(31):11742–7.
25. Cerdan C, Rouleau A, Bhatia M, et al. VEGF-A165 augments erythropoietic development from human embryonic stem cells. Blood 2004;103(7):2504–12.
26. Kennedy M, D'Souza SL, Lynch-Kattman M, et al. Development of the hemangioblast defines the onset of hematopoiesis in human ES cell differentiation cultures. Blood 2007;109(7):2679–87.
27. Zambidis ET, Peault B, Park TS, et al. Hematopoietic differentiation of human embryonic stem cells progresses through sequential hematoendothelial, primitive, and definitive stages resembling human yolk sac development. Blood 2005;106(3):860–70.
28. Chang KH, Nelson AM, Wang L, et al. Definitive-like erythroid cells derived from human embryonic stem cells coexpress high levels of embryonic and fetal globins with little or no adult globin. Blood 2006;108(5):1515–23.
29. Kaufman DS, Hanson ET, Lewis RL, et al. Hematopoietic colony-forming cells derived from human embryonic stem cells. Proc Natl Acad Sci U S A 2001; 98(19):10716–21.

30. Vodyanik MA, Bork JA, Thomson JA, et al. Human embryonic stem cell–derived CD34+ cells: efficient production in the coculture with OP9 stromal cells and analysis of lymphohematopoietic potential. Blood 2005;105(2):617–26.
31. Tian X, Morris JK, Linehan JL, et al. Cytokine requirements differ for stroma and embryoid body-mediated hematopoiesis from human embryonic stem cells. Exp Hematol 2004;32(10):1000–9.
32. Qiu C, Hanson E, Olivier E, et al. Differentiation of human embryonic stem cells into hematopoietic cells by coculture with human fetal liver cells recapitulates the globin switch that occurs early in development. Exp Hematol 2005;33(12):1450–8.
33. Vodyanik MA, Thomson JA, Slukvin II, et al. Leukosialin (CD43) defines hematopoietic progenitors in human embryonic stem cell differntiation cultures. Blood 2006;108(6):2095–105.
34. Olivier EN, Qiu C, Velho M, et al. Large-scale production of embryonic red blood cells from human embryonic stem cells. Exp Hematol 2006;34(12):1635–42.
35. Qiu C, Olivier EN, Velho M, et al. Globin switches in yolk sac-like primitive and fetal-like definitive red blood cells produced from human embryonic stem cells. Blood 2008;111(4):2400–8.
36. Carotta S, Pilat S, Mairhofer A, et al. Directed differentiation and mass cultivation of pure erythroid progenitors from mouse embryonic stem cells. Blood 2004;104(6):1873–80.
37. Jiang Y, Jahagirdar BN, Reinhardt RL, et al. Pluripotency of mesenchymal stem cells derived from adult marrow. Nature 2002;418(6893):41–9.
38. Kögler G, Sensken S, Airey JA, et al. A new human somatic stem cell from placental cord blood with intrinsic pluripotent differentiation potential. J Exp Med 2004;200(2):123–35.
39. De Coppi P, Bartsch G Jr, Siddiqui MM, et al. Isolation of amniotic stem cell lines with potential for therapy. Nat Biotechnol 2007;25(1):100–6.
40. Rideout WM 3rd, Hochedlinger K, Kyba M, et al. Correction of a genetic defect by nuclear transplantation and combined cell and gene therapy. Cellule 2002;109(1):17–27.
41. Takahashi K, Yamanaka S. Induction of pluripotent stem cells from mouse embryonic and adult fibroblast cultures by defined factors. Cellule 2006;126:663–76.
42. Okita K, Ichisaka T, Yamanaka S, et al. Generation of germline-competent induced pluripotent stem cells. Nature 2007;448(7151):313–7.
43. Wernig M, Meissner A, Foreman R, et al. In vitro reprogramming of fibroblasts into a pluripotent ES-cell-like state. Nature 2007;448(7151):318–24.
44. Park IH, Zhao R, West JA, et al. Reprogramming of human somatic cells to pluripotency with defined factors. Nature 2008;451(7175):141–6.
45. Takahashi K, Tanabe K, Ohnuki M, et al. Induction of pluripotent stem cells from adult human fibroblasts by defined factors. Cellule 2007;131(5):861–72.
46. Hanna J, Wernig M, Markoulaki S, et al. Treatment of sickle cell anemia mouse model with IPS cells generated from autologous skin. Science 2007;318(5858):1920–3.

Oxygen Therapeutics: Perfluorocarbons and Blood Substitute Safety

Claudia S. Cohn, MD, PhD[a], Melissa M. Cushing, MD[b],*

KEYWORDS

- Blood substitute • Perfluorocarbons (PFC)
- Hemoglobin-based-oxygen-carrier (HBOC)

The United States health care system depends on access to a blood supply that satisfies two important, but potentially conflicting, goals: safety and availability. Our donor-based system has demonstrated resilience in handling challenges as varied as seasonal shortages in supply to safety risks presented by emerging infectious diseases. Although we can be confident in future innovations in blood supply management, the aging United States population will present twin challenges to our system. First, as procedure volumes increase to care for senior citizens, demand for blood components will increase. Second, the availability of blood components could be challenged as the donor pool shrinks; younger generations have yet to demonstrate the altruism of blood donation shown by their forebears.

Although the need for a blood substitute has become more urgent, the clinical usefulness of blood substitutes has encouraged centuries of exploration. Early recorded efforts included the use of milk and wine as blood substitutes. The use of animal blood in transfusions was explored more recently with no success.[1–3] Subsequent initiatives led by the military (seeking a battlefield solution to blood loss) and the private sector (recognizing the risk of HIV to the blood supply) have focused on two general categories of oxygen carriers: perfluorocarbons (PFCs) and hemoglobin-based oxygen carriers (HBOCs). PFCs are completely synthetic, whereas HBOCs are made from human or animal-derived hemoglobin (Hb). Other products, such as recombinant Hb, are in preclinical development. Several of these oxygen carriers are undergoing clinical trials; however, many prior attempts have resulted in adverse events and have been discontinued.

[a] Department of Pathology, New York Presbyterian Hospital/Weill-Cornell, 525 East 68th Street, Room F-710, New York, NY 10065, USA
[b] Department of Pathology, Weill Cornell Medical College, 525 East 68th Street, Room F-544A, New York, NY 10065, USA
* Corresponding author.
E-mail address: mec2013@med.cornell.edu (M.M. Cushing).

Crit Care Clin 25 (2009) 399–414
doi:10.1016/j.ccc.2008.12.007   criticalcare.theclinics.com
0749-0704/08/$ – see front matter © 2009 Elsevier Inc. All rights reserved.

It is important to differentiate between "blood substitutes" and "red cell substitutes." Red cell substitutes are oxygen carriers and do not replace all components and functions of blood (coagulation factors and white blood cells).

At the time of this writing, the many functions of human red blood cells have no true substitute and the authors do not believe that blood substitutes will replace the need for blood donation in the foreseeable future. Over time and with improvements, they believe that these technologies have the potential to dramatically reshape the practice of transfusion medicine. In this article, the authors define the attributes of an ideal blood substitute (**Box 1**), discuss the history, mechanism, and current status of PFCs, and review the shortcomings of all oxygen therapeutic products in development today.

MEETING THE NEED: THE IDEAL BLOOD SUBSTITUTE

The ideal blood substitute would answer the challenges of safety and availability (see **Box 1**). To ensure safety, the ideal blood substitute would reduce disease transmission and immunosuppressive effects while enhancing oxygen delivery. To improve availability, the ideal blood substitute would be eligible for cost-effective mass production, universal compatibility, prolonged shelf life, and ease of administration. As an added clinical benefit, blood substitutes could address some medical needs in a better fashion than intact red cells.

Many attempts have been made to develop blood substitutes under the current regulatory structure, but no product has been able to fulfill all of the above criteria or meet the Food and Drug Administration's (FDA's) requirements of purity, potency, and safety. The unmet clinical need has inspired several companies to continue to research red cell substitutes and fund preclinical development and clinical trials.

Box 1
Characteristics of an ideal blood substitute

No risk of disease transmission

No immunosuppressive effects

No interaction with the immune system

Maintenance of arterial blood pressure and pH

Availability of abundant supply

Universal compatibility (no need to type and crossmatch)

Rapid metabolization and elimination in vivo

Prolonged shelf life and stability at a range of temperatures

In vivo half-life similar to the red blood cell

Similar viscosity to blood

Availability at a reasonable cost

Ease of administering

Ability to access all areas of the human body (including ischemic tissue)

No interference with capillary circulation

Effectiveness at room air or ambient conditions

PERFLUOROCARBONS: MECHANISM OF ACTION AND HISTORY

PFCs are synthetic compounds made of fluorine atoms replacing hydrogen atoms along an 8-10 molecule carbon backbone. The replacement of hydrogen with fluorine yields a rigid molecule with a dense electronic sheath that gives a "Scotch-guard like effect" at the molecular level.[4] PFCs are highly hydrophobic and lipophobic, and are chemically inert compounds that cannot be metabolized in vivo. They are immiscible in water and can dissolve gases such as oxygen and carbon dioxide better than any other liquid because of their intrinsic molecular structure. Because PFCs carry oxygen by direct solubility, their contribution to oxygen content is directly proportional to the arterial oxygen tension (PaO_2) and requires a high PaO_2 (>300 mm Hg) to be effective, unlike Hb, which covalently binds and releases oxygen in a cooperative manner, yielding a sinusoidal, rather than a linear, dissociation curve (**Fig. 1**). The combination of biologic inertness with superior oxygen and carbon dioxide solubilities promotes the concept of PFC as a viable red blood cell substitute.

In 1966, Leland C. Clark[5] submerged a mouse for several hours in an oxygenated PFC. Although the mouse later died of lung injury, this experiment launched an intensive effort to bring PFCs from the bench to the bedside. Several technical problems were defined during this early period. An ideal PFC must be "heavy enough" to be emulsified for injection, but also "light enough" to be lipid soluble for rapid excretion. It must also be optimized for vapor pressure, to avoid retention of air in the alveoli, which causes increased pulmonary residual volume. PFC emulsions are produced by high shear homogenization of small PFC droplets with egg yolk phospholipids. The emulsion is terminally heat sterilized and adjusted for pH and osmolarity.

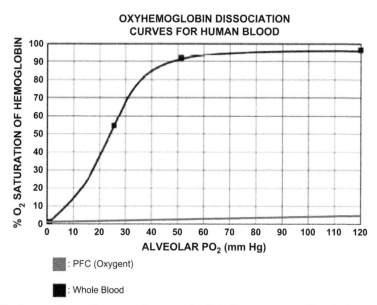

OXYHEMOGLOBIN DISSOCIATION CURVES FOR HUMAN BLOOD

■ : PFC (Oxygent)

■ : Whole Blood

Fig. 1. Perfluorocarbons demonstrate a nearly flat, linear oxygen dissociation curve in contrast to the sigmoidal dissociation curve of hemoglobin. As a result, most of the oxygen bound to PFCs is released in the high pressure atmosphere of the arteries, with little bound oxygen available for the capillary network where the partial pressure of oxygen is lower, and hence the need for oxygen is greater.

First Commercial Application of Perfluorocarbons

The first PFC developed commercially was Fluosol-DA (Green Cross Corp., Osaka, Japan), using the PFC perfluorodecalin in an albumin emulsion. Fluosol-DA contained only 10% PFC by volume and was stored frozen. An early clinical trial of Fluosol-DA tested its safety and efficacy in acute anemia. Twenty-three surgical patients who had blood loss and religious objections to receiving blood transfusions were evaluated. Although no serious adverse reactions were noted, no appreciable beneficial effects of Fluosol-DA were seen.[6] A newer formulation by Alpha Therapeutics (Grifols USA, Los Angeles, California) led to FDA approval of Fluosol in 1989 for use in high-risk coronary balloon angioplasty. It holds the distinction of being the only oxygen therapeutic to be approved for human clinical use in the United States. Fluosol suffered from multiple clinical shortcomings, however, which led to its removal from the market in 1994. First, Fluosol delivered only 0.4 mL oxygen per 100 mL, requiring patients to receive supplemental oxygen. Because the oxygen was unloaded in a manner linear with PaO_2, most of the oxygen was released before arrival at the microvasculature, where it was most needed. Second, Fluosol was excreted slowly and some metabolites remained in the body for months. Third, Fluosol had biologic side effects, including a temporary decrease in platelet count and flu-like symptoms (myalgia and fever). These symptoms were thought to occur because PFC particle droplets were large enough to activate macrophages, which released proinflammatory cytokines.[7] Finally, Fluosol had short product stability (8 hours) after reconstitution, which created logistical difficulties during angioplasties.

Second-Generation Perfluorocarbons

With lessons learned from Fluosol and other early PFC developments, several companies developed a second generation of PFC emulsions. Notable changes included a high PFC content, which theoretically reduced the absolute requirement for the maintenance of a fraction of inspired oxygen (FIO_2) greater than 0.8 (as with Fluosol-DA) for optimal efficacy. The second-generation PFC could also be removed from the blood by plasmapheresis, making intraoperative use more feasible. Finally, this product could be given with autologous blood transfusions. Four second-generation PFCs were developed: Oxygent, Oxycyte, Oxyfluor, and Perftoran (which has not undergone clinical review in the United States).

Oxygent (Alliance Corp., San Diego, California) is an improved second-generation concentrated PFC emulsion composed primarily of perflubron (perfluorooctyl bromide; $C_8F_{17}Br$), with a small percentage of F-decyl bromide added to maintain small droplet size and thus eliminate macrophage activation. The addition of F-decyl bromide also prevents excessive organ retention of the PFC. Oxygent has a shelf life of 2 years when stored at 4°C, and is ready for use. It still requires oxygen inhalation by the patient, however, because the oxygen delivery capacity is less than 30% of normal blood.[8]

A large European multicenter phase III study has shown that Oxygent, in conjunction with acute normovolemic hemodilution, reduced the need for red blood cell transfusion in 492 patients undergoing major noncardiac surgery.[9] The patients were randomly distributed into two groups. The control group was transfused intraoperatively at an Hb concentration of less than 8.0 g/dL. The PFC-treated patients first underwent acute normovolemic hemodilution to Hb of 8.0 g/dL, followed by dosing with Oxygent. The patients receiving Oxygent had a significant reduction in the number of packed red blood cells transfused throughout their hospital stay when compared with the control group (26% versus 16%; $P<.05$). However, more serious adverse events were reported in the PFC group (32%) than in controls (21%; $P<.05$).

A second phase III trial studying Oxygent in patients undergoing cardiopulmonary bypass was terminated in the United States because of a possible increase in stroke rates in the Oxygent treatment arm. Unfortunately, studies on this product have been halted because of development costs, suggesting that those familiar with the product were not confident in its clinical or commercial success.[10]

Oxyfluor (HemaGen, Sunset Hills, Missouri) consists of perfluorodichlorooctane in an emulsion. Its advantages include a significantly higher oxygen delivery capacity than Fluosol, and extended stability at room temperature. Preclinical studies indicated that it did not cause pulmonary hyperinflation and was readily eliminated from the lung, liver, and spleen. Early-phase clinical trials were successfully completed with only mild thrombocytopenia and flu-like symptoms reported in healthy human volunteers. Dose escalation studies were planned; however, a major financial backer, Baxter International, withdrew support, ending development of this product.[11]

Oxycyte (Synthetic Blood International, Costa Mesa, California) is composed of the $C_{10}F_{20}$ PFC emulsified in water for injection with purified egg yolk phospholipids. In Phase II clinical trials, Oxycyte was tested in patients who had traumatic brain injury. Although no published data are available from this trial, the company stated that the primary end point of increasing patients' PaO_2 levels compared with baseline was met. A second phase II trial was suspended for this product.

Perftoran (Perftoran, Pushchino, Russia) contains perfluorodecalin and perfluoro-N-(4-methylcyclohexyl)-piperidine emulsified by the nonionic surfactant Proxanol-268. Perftoran can be stored frozen for 3 years or at $4°C$ for 2 weeks. Perftoran has been widely used in Russia, with more than 3000 patients treated in comparative studies. Indications have included acute blood loss and hemorrhagic shock, occlusion of blood vessels and acute myocardial infarct, transplantation, and local application for wounds and ulcers. Perftoran was also used to prevent ischemia in cadaveric kidneys awaiting transplant.[12] In these studies, Perftoran was sometimes used with a combination of plasma expanders while supplemental oxygen was given. Adverse reactions such as hypotension and pulmonary complications were observed during massive blood replacement with Perftoran in about 1% of cases.

In a randomized clinical trial of Perftoran in Mexico City, Mexico, 30 patients scheduled for elective cardiac valvuloplasty surgery were randomly divided into a treatment and control arm. The Perftoran group had significantly higher intraoperative PaO_2 levels and needed fewer allogeneic red blood cell packs than the control group.[13] No complications or deaths were reported in either group. This small study is the sole example of a published, controlled clinical trial using Perftoran. Until a well-designed clinical trial is performed, it is unlikely that Perftoran will be widely adopted.

Outlook for Perfluorocarbons

At the current time, no clinical trials are ongoing in the United States with a PFC as a blood substitute (**Table 1**). Although Perftoran is used in Russia and Mexico, because of the lack of clinical evidence in the United States and the timeline for FDA approval, Perftoran is unlikely to be used in the United States in the near future. In their current state, PFCs do not appear to be a likely technology platform for a viable blood substitute. The in vivo use of the PFC Perflubron (Alliance Pharmaceuticals, San Diego, California) as a contrast agent for MRI has FDA approval.

Table 1. Perfluorocarbons

Name (Manufacturer)	Composition	Clinical Studies	Associated Adverse Effects	Other
Fluosol-DA (Green Cross)	Perfluorodecalin	Phase III	Flu-like symptoms; Transient decrease in platelet levels	FDA approval in 1989 for balloon angioplasty; Removed from market in 1994
Oxygent (Alliance)	Perflubron with F-decyl bromide	Phase III	Increase in stroke rates	—
Oxyfluor (HemaGen)	Perfluorodichlorooctane	Phase I, Ib, and II	Flu-like symptoms; Transient decrease in platelet levels	—
Oxycyte (Synthetic Blood Intl.)	$C_{10}F_{20}$	Phase II	No data available	No published data
Perftoran (Perftoran)	Perfluorodecalin/perfluoro-N-(4-methylcyclohexyl)-piperidine	Randomized trial in Mexico City	Hypotension; Pulmonary complications	In use in Russia and Mexico

TOXICITY, SAFETY, AND INTERFERENCE IN BLOOD SUBSTITUTES
Toxicities

The toxicities associated with PFCs are minimal, likely because of their composition. When used as blood substitutes, some mild immunologic effects, such as macrophage activation leading to flu-like symptoms, have been reported. Yet in MRI procedures, patients ingest large volumes of Perflubron with little ill effect (diarrhea is the most common adverse effect). The safety of Hb-based red cell substitutes, however, remains uncertain (**Table 2**). Although cross-linking and polymerizing Hb subunits have reduced the incidence of nephrotoxicity, problems with vasoconstriction, direct Hb-mediated cytotoxicity, immune-mediated cytokine stimulation, and altered immune function are potential concerns. The associated toxicities can be broadly grouped into four categories: neurovascular, immunologic, gastrointestinal, and infectious.

Neurovascular

Vasoactivity
Most common among the problems associated with HBOCs is vasoconstriction with subsequent hypertension. The primary mechanism is likely the binding of nitric oxide to Hb. Free Hb is a known nitric oxide scavenger. The free Hb within HBOCs can leak through the vascular endothelium and scavenge the sequestered nitric oxide. Nitric oxide mediates smooth muscle relaxation by inhibiting the conversion of proendothelin to endothelin, a potent vasoconstrictor. When nitric oxide binds Hb, endothelin is produced, causing increases in systemic and pulmonary arterial pressures and vascular resistance. Polyheme, a polymerized HBOC, has not caused any problems with vasoconstriction, perhaps because the polymers of Hb do not extravasate and subsequently bind nitric oxide in the endothelium.[14]

Other mechanisms are likely at work. HBOCs with low oxygen affinity and PFCs that unload oxygen in a linear manner can cause excessive tissue oxygenation, which can lead to reflex vasoconstriction, an increase in systemic blood pressure, a decrease in heart rate and a concomitant decrease in cardiac output. This scenario was seen with intramolecular cross-linked hemoglobin ($\alpha\alpha$-Hb, Baxter Healthcare, Deerfield, Illinois), and a recombinant analog, rHb1.1 (Somatogen Inc., Boulder, Colorado). These

Table 2
Toxicities of oxygen therapeutics

Description	Products Involved	Hypothetic/Reported
Neurovascular		
Neurotoxicity	HBOC	Reported[16–18]
Vasoactivity	HBOC	Reported[14,15]
Immunologic		
Immunogenicity	HBOC	Hypothetic
Altered immune function	PFC, HBOC/Liposome	Reported[7,19,20]
Gastrointestinal		
Gastrointestinal complaints	HBOC	Reported[21]
Pancreatitis	HBOC	Reported[22–25]
Infectious		
Sepsis	HBOC	Hypothetic
Prion risk	Bovine-derived HBOC	Hypothetic

products were intensely vasoconstrictive in preclinical and clinical studies and ultimately abandoned.[15]

Neurotoxicity

The blood–brain barrier can be disrupted during traumatic head injury, stroke, and subarachnoid hemorrhage. If patients are treated with HBOC, the potentially toxic effect of free Hb on neurons should be known. Studies have been performed to evaluate various HBOCs' effects on cerebral blood flow and neuronal toxicity. In vitro testing of stroma-free Hb showed that Hb killed neurons while leaving glial cells intact.[16] Other researchers however, working with HBOC-201, found that it was not toxic to neural cells in culture.[17] A third study evaluated the effects of diaspirin cross-linked hemoglobin (DCLHb, Baxter Healthcare) given after subarachnoid hemorrhage in rats. Although DCLHb did decrease cerebral blood flow more than a "mock cerebral fluid" but less than autologous blood did, fewer dead neurons were found in the DCLHb-treated group.[18] The contradicting data from these studies may be due to differences in methodology and blood product tested.

Immunologic

Immunogenicity

Because modified human Hb has been chemically changed, it may be possible for it to trigger an immune response in humans. Bovine Hb has an even greater chance of causing immunogenicity in humans because of substantial differences in the protein structure of bovine and human Hbs. To date, no serious immune or allergic responses have been reported, but most patients have only had single incident exposures to these products, usually over short periods of time. Animal studies by manufacturers have not demonstrated a problem.

Altered immune function

PFCs, liposome-encapsulated Hbs, and HBOCs can stimulate or suppress the immune system, causing adverse events. As discussed above (see PFC overview), the particle size of first-generation PFCs caused production of cytokines by activated macrophages, which led to the complaint of flu-like symptoms in treated patients and a transient decrease in platelet counts. Impaired neutrophil function has also been noted.[19] An in vitro study showed that PFC was selectively cytotoxic to macrophages.[7]

Liposome-encapsulated Hbs and HBOCs can activate the reticuloendothelial system and the complement and coagulation pathways, and can cause platelet aggregation. These activities are mediated by nitric oxide scavenging and can cause hepatosplenomegaly.[20]

Gastrointestinal

Gastrointestinal complaints

Clinical findings of abdominal discomfort, pain, nausea, and vomiting have been reported with HBOC administration. Hb interaction and scavenging of nitric oxide is also thought to play a role in some gastrointestinal effects of the products. Nitric oxide is believed to be required for relaxation of the lower esophageal sphincter during swallowing. In animal and human subjects, intravenous infusion with HBOC has caused dysphagia.[21] It has also been hypothesized that increases in pancreatic enzymes, such as amylase and lipase, result from scavenging of nitric oxide resulting in spasms of the Sphincter of Oddi.

Pancreatitis

Pancreatitis has been reported as an adverse event in three HBOC clinical trials, affecting 17 treated patients versus three control patients. The pathophysiology underlying these data may be multifaceted. Many studies have linked ischemia and acute pancreatitis;[22] however, when researchers tried to show that vasoconstriction caused by HBOC scavenging of nitric oxide played a role in acute pancreatitis, no causal relationship could be proved.

Stronger data support the link between HBOC production of reactive oxygen species and acute pancreatitis. Stroma-free Hb and its metabolites, free iron and heme, can produce oxygen-free radicals that may cause free radical injury in tissues,[23] which can lead to oxidative stress in the pancreas and contribute to the development and progression of acute pancreatitis.[24,25]

Hematologic

Hematologic effects

A randomized, single-dose study of HBOC-201 found that serum iron, ferritin, and erythropoietin levels increased in healthy volunteers. The erythropoietin levels were elevated twofold to sixfold over baseline.[20] Although elevations of iron and ferritin may be beneficial in severely anemic patients, care must be taken to avoid iron overload in chronically transfused patient populations (eg, thalassemics).

An additional HBOC-related toxicity may result from the rate at which HBOC products are oxidized to methemoglobin, which could limit prolonged or high doses of HBOCs. When products were measured on various instruments, methemoglobin levels in Hemolink (Hemosol BioPharma Inc, Mississauga, Ontario, Canada), DCLHb, and rHb 1.1 were all elevated (up to 24.9% in one product).[26] However, methemoglobin levels have not reached pathologic concentrations in vivo in either animal or human HBOC trials.[27]

Infectious

Sepsis

The complications of red cell substitutes in septic patients are not known. Cell-free Hb substances may support bacterial virulence by offering a ready supply of iron, thus sustaining bacterial replication and inhibiting neutrophil function. Although animal data have been suggestive of a potential clinical problem, clinical trials to date have not established this risk.[28]

Prions

The risk for contracting Creutzfeldt-Jakob Disease (CJD) from bovine-derived HBOC products (eg, Hemopure, Biopure Corp., Cambridge, Massachusetts) creates additional safety hurdles for these products. In the late 1990s, scientists discovered that a new variant of CJD could be transmitted from cattle to humans through the ingestion of cow brain and spinal cord material,[29] which led the FDA to prohibit the transfusion of blood products from donors who spent extended periods of time in the United Kingdom. Although Biopure scientists have published studies showing that viruses and "transmissible spongiform encephalopathy agents" (the prion protein underlying CJD) can be cleared from their products,[30] further experimental studies and long-term epidemiologic monitoring are warranted.[31]

TESTING INTERFERENCE

Interference of PFCs and HBOCs on some routine laboratory tests could be a serious problem, especially if these products become available for mainstream use. Because the composition of these products differs dramatically, so too does the nature of their interference (**Table 3**). Although each commercially available PFC differs slightly in PFC content and emulsifying agent, HBOCs have dramatic differences. Each product may produce a unique and characteristic interference profile; however, published studies are limited.

PERFLUOROCARBON INTERFERENCE

CO-oximeters are multiwavelength spectrophotometers that measure the optical absorbance of blood at different wavelengths and automatically calculate the fractional concentration of the four major Hb species (oxy-, deoxy-, carboxy-, and methemoglobin) from a total Hb concentration. PFCs have been shown to interfere with CO-oximetry testing. When perflubron was added to standardized blood samples, it adversely affected some of the hemolyzing CO-oximeters but did not interfere with nonhemolyzing instruments. The hemolyzing CO-oximeters experienced concentration-dependent interference in their measurement of all analytes except total Hb concentration.[32]

The second-generation PFC Oxyfluor generated spurious elevations in platelet counts in vitro, which was attributed to the emulsion particles being counted as platelets by automated hematology analyzers, resulting in reproducible overestimates of the platelet counts.[33] PFCs have also been shown to interfere negatively with the analysis of amylase and plasma iron, and interfere positively with ammonia and phosphorus. The positive phosphorus interference is caused by the phosphate-buffered saline content in the Perflubron emulsion.[34]

Despite the fact that blood containing PFCs emulsions can have a lipemic appearance, the common laboratory interference problems associated with lipemic light scattering have not been reported. When lipemic interference was tested, a 1:20 dilution of Perflubron in plasma produced a "lipemic index" of 35. This value was well below the lower limit of 50 programmed in some instruments to produce an alert flag for a patient's sample.[34]

HEMOGLOBIN-BASED-OXYGEN-CARRIER INTERFERENCE
Interference Related to Free Hemoglobin

The mechanisms underlying testing interference with HBOCs are largely related to the presence of free Hb. The soluble Hb imparts a red/hemolyzed appearance to a patient's plasma, which could lead to false alarms among untrained medical personnel. The Hb from HBOCs will also distort the canonical 3:1 rule between hematocrit and Hb, commonly used to judge blood's oxygen-carrying capacity from hematocrit. Clinical laboratories must also be aware of HBOC usage because Hb

Table 3 Laboratory interferences encountered with blood substitutes		
Method	PFC	HBOC
CO-oximetry	+	+
Clot-based assays	−	+
Spectrophotometry	±	+++
Pretransfusion testing	?	−

species have a strong optical absorbance between 500 and 600 nm, which can cause interference in many colorimetric and spectrophotometric methods used.[34]

Like PFCs, HBOCs can perturb CO-oximetry measurements. A study using five HBOCS (DCLHb; Oxyglobin, Biopure; ApexPHP, Apex Bioscience, Research Triangle Park, North Carolina; Hemolink; and rHb1.1 (Somatogen Inc.), Hb Therapeutics/Baxter Healthcare) and eight CO-oximeters found varying levels of interference with all HBOCs tested. The interference occurred with measurements of all four major Hb species. The findings of interference with bovine-derived Oxyglobin (an HBOC used in veterinary medicine) held up even when the optical extinction coefficient for bovine Hb was used.[26]

Interference with Optical-Based Methods

The effect of various HBOCs on the coagulation system and coagulation testing has been studied.[35-37] The results of these studies have varied widely, with each product reacting differently in different assays. Using alternatives to optical-based clot-detection methods alleviated interference problems.[35,38] Shirey and colleagues[38] studied the effect of the presence of HBOC on pretransfusion testing and found that HBOC did not interfere with results when standard methods were used.

Most chemistry tests using photometric methods suffer because of interference from HBOCs. Multiple studies examined common analyte measurements in the presence of varying concentrations of HBOCs. Two studies used different analyzers to gauge the interference created by HBOCs from Biopure. These studies found variable interferences when testing albumin, alkaline phosphatase, amylase, alanine aminotransferase, aspartate aminotransferase, bilirubin (total and conjugated), calcium, cholesterol, gamma glutamyl transpeptidase, lactate dehydrogenase, lipase, phosphate, and total protein.[34,39-41] The assays monitored reaction rates bichromatically and were designed to detect hemolysis and other sources of interference. They were not capable of correcting for the higher concentrations of Hb present in HBOC samples. These studies also found interference with gentamicin and vancomycin measurements, which are not photometric-based assays, suggesting other types of interference are present.[41] In addition, creatinine measurements showed interference; however, simple filtration of the samples resolved this problem.

The interference with lactate measurement caused by Oxyglobin, Hemopure, and Hemolink has also been assessed. Combinations of L-lactate, HBOC, and blood or plasma were used, with lactate concentrations ranging from 5 to 110 mg/dL (0.6–12 mm). As HBOC levels increased in plasma, lactate measurements became increasingly inaccurate, especially at larger lactate concentrations. Interference caused the lactate values to be underestimated.[42]

Hemoglobin Vesicles Interference

These Hbs encapsulated within a phospholipid bilayer membrane were found to cause serious interference in most of the 30 analytes studied. The interference was greater than that seen with soluble acellular Hb solution. Simple ultracentrifugation proved to be the solution used to alleviate interference with Hb-containing vesicles. By centrifuging a serum preparation containing Hb vesicles at 50,000 × the force of gravity for 20 minutes and removing the Hb vesicles precipitate, the interference was eliminated. A similar method could not be used with HBOCs.[43]

Safety

The safety of blood substitutes must be measured against the risks inherent in blood transfusions or the morbidity/mortality associated with receiving no transfusion at all.

The complications of blood transfusions include transfusion reactions, alloimmuniza-tion, and disease transmission. For blood substitutes to be used routinely, the risk for an adverse event must be, at most, comparable to these risks. In addition, for patients who cannot receive blood, because of either religious beliefs or locale, the risk of a blood substitute must be compared with the risk of inaction or use of plasma expanders.

One safety issue involves the use of bovine Hb to produce some HBOC products. Bovine Hb was sought as an alternative to human Hb because it has naturally low oxygen affinity and can be directly polymerized (to avoid renal excretion) without prior manipulation. Other advantages include bovine Hb's molecular structure, which has enhanced oxygen unloading in ischemic tissue. Unlike human Hb, which is regulated by 2,3-diphosphoglycerate, the affinity of bovine Hb is partially regulated by serum chloride ions.[44] Although this product removes the constraint of using human-donated red blood cells, uncertainties exist about using bovine Hb because of its potential to transmit disease (see above discussion of prions) and its potential immunogenicity.

To approve a blood substitute for commercial use, the FDA requires demonstration of safety and clinical benefit. Although clinical benefit of a substitute may be difficult to demonstrate given the efficacy of blood, safety should be clearly demonstrable. A report compiled by the FDA summarizes the adverse events from eight clinical trials of HBOCs that were reported in the literature or publicly available.[25] In the categories of death, myocardial infarction, and cerebrovascular accident/ischemia/transient ischemic event, the treated cohort outnumbered the control arm by ~2:1. The treated group also suffered from a greater number of less severe adverse events compared with the control group.

A recent meta-analysis of Hb-based blood substitutes used in surgical, stroke, and trauma patients examined the data on death and myocardial infarction as outcome variables in 16 clinical trials.[45] The products studied included HemAssist (Baxter Healthcare); Hemopure; Hemolink; PolyHeme (Northfield Laboratories Inc., Evanston, Illinois); and Hemospan (Sangart Inc., San Diego, California). Based on the analysis of available data, the investigators found a 30% increase in the risk for death and a 2.7-fold increase in the risk for myocardial infarction when all HBOC trials were pooled. Subgroup analyses of these trials indicated that the increased risk was not restricted to a particular HBOC or clinical indication, although the investigators pointed out that these analyses had reduced statistical power. Based on the findings in this report, and preclinical evidence of potential toxicity for the HBOCs reviewed, a recent editorial recommended the cessation of further HBOC phase III trials.[46]

The data in the above meta-analysis also brought to light the importance of timely reporting of study results to the FDA. According to their review, if a prompt meta-anal-ysis of the cumulative data had been performed by 2000, when several studies had already been concluded, then multiple product-related deaths and myocardial infarcts could have been avoided. New technologies can bring equal parts promise and peril; therefore, strict adherence to safety guidelines is necessary to tip the balance toward positive progress.

Although the widespread clinical use of these technologies as blood substitutes in the United States appears limited, a potential application may still be in demand on the battlefield. The FDA has approved avoidance of transfusion as an end point for red cell substitute clinical trials. Thus, the trials involving these products have naturally gravi-tated to clinical situations, such as trauma, where an acute situation of hemorrhage exists in an underlying healthy individual who is capable of recovering his or her own red cell mass and function.

SUMMARY

Current concerns over the blood supply in developed and developing countries will compound over time. Emerging infectious diseases, such as dengue, avian influenza virus, and chikungunya virus, present additional safety risks to our blood supply. The demographic tidal wave of an aging population will squeeze supply levels; demand for blood products will increase at the same time as an aging donor base is replaced by successor generations who have not demonstrated the blood donation altruism of their elders.

Red cell substitutes have a promising value proposition for transfusion services: Increase the availability of blood products and remove donor and contamination safety risks. Can substitutes deliver on their promise? Will issues of safety and toxicity overwhelm the industry?

This article has highlighted the challenge of clinical approval. Existing products suffer from critical shortcomings (eg, vasoactivity) that make them more suitable for short-term gaps (eg, acute blood loss, ischemia, bridge until compatible red cells become available) than long-term solutions. Substitutes not based on human blood introduce potentially more complex safety hurdles, such as immunogenicity and fear of prion contamination in bovine-derived products.

The FDA needs to maximize its leadership position and strengthen the safety criteria for clinical trials for these products to be credible and marketable to the medical community. Even if safety and toxicity problems are overcome, blood substitutes will only have a niche application unless they can be produced in meaningful volume and provided at a reasonable price. Given the substantial investment required for clinical approval, it is likely that the first available substitutes will be expensive. Although market forces will eventually determine a price equilibrium, it is likely to take time for substitutes to be as cost effective as human red blood cells.

When a product becomes available in this country, certain implementation questions are bound to surface. Where should the red cell substitutes be stored in the hospital: the blood bank or the pharmacy? Would community blood centers need to increase collections to facilitate the manufacture of HBOC? How should their use be prioritized in view of the likelihood of limited supplies? Could certain potential donors who are currently deferred provide red cells for pathogen-inactivated Hb solutions? Should oxygen therapeutics be considered part of a strategic blood reserve in case of terrorist attacks or other national disasters?

The true impact of red blood cell substitutes is not yet known. Will the current safety issues obscure their potential use? Will a new generation of HBOCs or PFCs emerge as new technologies develop? This article suggests that we are several years from knowing the answer to these questions. Until significant changes occur, the transfusion community needs to redouble its efforts to enhance the blood supply while still applying stringent standards for safety and efficacy to new products.

REFERENCES

1. Amberson WR, Mulder AG, Steggerda FR, et al. Mammalian life without red blood corpuscles. Science 1933;78:106–7.
2. Brandt JL, Frank NR, Lichtman HC, et al. The effects of hemoglobin solutions on renal functions in man. Blood 1951;6:1152–8.
3. Miller JH, McDonald RK. The effect of hemoglobin on renal function in the human. J Clin Invest 1951;30:1033–40.

4. Riess JG. Understanding the fundamentals of perfluorocarbons and perfluorocarbon emulsions relevant to in vivo oxygen delivery. Artif Cells Blood Substit Immobil Biotechnol 2005;33:47–63.

5. Clark LC Jr, Gollan F. Survival of mammals breathing organic liquids equilibrated with oxygen at atmospheric pressure. Science 1966;152:1755–6.

6. Gould SA, Rosen AL, Sehgal LR, et al. Fluosol-DA as a red-cell substitute in acute anemia. N Engl J Med 1986;314:1653–6.

7. Bucala R, Kawakami M, Cerami A, et al. Cytotoxicity of a perfluorocarbon blood substitute to macrophages in vitro. Science 1983;220:965–7.

8. Riess JG. Perfluorocarbon-based oxygen delivery. Artif Cells Blood Substit Immobil Biotechnol 2006;34:567–80.

9. Spahn DR, Waschke KF, Standl T, et al. Use of perflubron emulsion to decrease allogeneic blood transfusion in high-blood-loss non-cardiac surgery: results of a European phase 3 study. Anesthesiology 2002;97:1338–49.

10. Niiler E. Setbacks for blood substitute companies. Nat Biotechnol 2002;20:962–3.

11. Riess JG, Krafft MP. Fluorocarbon emulsions as in vivo oxygen delivery systems: background and chemistry. In: Winslow RM, editor. Blood substitutes. 1st edition. New York: Academic Press; 2006. p. 259–76.

12. Maevsky E, Ivanitsky G, Bogdanova L, et al. Clinical results of perftoran application: present and future. Artif Cells Blood Substit Immobil Biotechnol 2005;33:37–46.

13. Verdin-Vasquez RC, Zepeda-Perez C, Ferra-Ferrer R, et al. Use of perftoran emulsion to decrease allogeneic blood transfusion in cardiac surgery: clinical trial. Artif Cells Blood Substit Immobil Biotechnol 2006;34:433–54.

14. Hess JR, MacDonald VW, Brinkley WW, et al. Systemic and pulmonary hypertension after resuscitation with cell-free hemoglobin. J Appl Phys 1993;74:1769–78.

15. Hess JR. Blood substitutes for surgery and trauma: efficacy and toxicity issues. BioDrugs 1999;12:81–90.

16. Ortegon DP, Davis MR, Dixon PS, et al. The polymerized bovine hemoglobin-based oxygen-carrying solution (HBOC-201) is not toxic to neural cells in culture. J Trauma 2002;53:1068–72.

17. Cole DJ, Nary JC, Reynolds LW, et al. Experimental subarachnoid hemorrhage in rats: effect of intravenous alpha-alpha diaspirin crosslinked hemoglobin on hypoperfusion and neuronal death. Anesthesiology 1997;87:1486–93.

18. Kim HW, Greenburg AG. Artificial oxygen carriers as red blood cell substitutes: a selected review and current status. Artif Organs 2004;28:813–28.

19. Winslow RM. Current status of oxygen carriers ('blood substitutes'): 2006. Vox Sang 2006;91:102–10.

20. Hughes GS Jr, Francome SF, Antal EJ, et al. Hematologic effects of a novel hemoglobin-based oxygen carrier in normal male and female subjects. J Lab Clin Med 1995;126:444–51.

21. Jahr JS, Walker V, Manoochehri K, et al. Blood substitutes as pharmacotherapies in clinical practice. Curr Opin Anaesthesiol 2007;20:325–30.

22. Warshaw AL, O'Hara PJ. Susceptibility of the pancreas to ischemic injury in shock. Ann Surg 1978;188:197–201.

23. Henkel-Honke T, Oleck M. Artificial oxygen carriers: a current review. AANA J 2007;75:205–11.

24. Kleinhans H, Mann O, Schurr PG, et al. Oxygen radical formation does not have an impact in the treatment of severe acute experimental pancreatitis using free cellular hemoglobin. World J Gastroenterol 2006;12:2914–8.

25. Silverman T, Landow L, Ko HS. et al. Review of publicly available reports of adverse events associated with HBOCs. Office of Blood Research and Review, CBER, FDA. 2008.

26. Ali AA, Ali GS, Steinke JM, et al. Co-oximetry interference by hemoglobin-based blood substitutes. Anesth Analg 2001;92:863–9.

27. Griffiths E, Cortes A, Gilbert N, et al. Haemoglobin-based blood substitutes and sepsis. Lancet 1995;345:158–60.

28. Will RG, Ironside JW, Zeidler M, et al. A new variant of Creutzfeldt-Jakob disease in the UK. Lancet 1996;347:921–5.

29. Laccetti A, Bagai J, Gawryl MS, et al. Hemopure's process demonstrates TSE and viral clearance. Dev Biol (Basel) 2005;120:35–6.

30. Burdick MD, Pifat DY, Petteway SR Jr, et al. Clearance of prions during plasma protein manufacture. Transfus Med Rev 2006;20:57–62.

31. Shepherd AP, Steinke JM. Co-oximetry interference by perflubron emulsion: comparison of hemolyzing and nonhemolyzing instruments. Clin Chem 1998; 44:2183–90.

32. Cuignet OY, Wood BL, Chandler WL, et al. A second-generation blood substitute (perfluorodichlorooctane emulsion) generates spurious elevations in platelet counts from automated hematology analyzers. Anesth Analg 2000;90:517–22.

33. Ma Z, Monk TG, Goodnough LT, et al. Effect of hemoglobin- and perflubron-based oxygen carriers on common clinical laboratory tests. Clin Chem 1997; 43:1732–7.

34. Moreira PL, Lansden CC, Clark TL, et al. Effect of Hemopure on prothrombin time and activated partial thromboplastin time on seven coagulation analyzers. Clin Chem 1997;43:1792.

35. Leytin V, Mazer D, Mody M, et al. Hemolink, an o-raffinose cross-linked haemo-globin-based oxygen carrier, does not affect activation and function of human platelets in whole blood in vitro. Br J Haematol 2003;120:535–41.

36. James MF, Potgieter HE, Ellis P, et al. The effect of Hemopure on coagulation in clinically relevant concentrations. Anesth Analg 2004;99:1593–7, table of contents.

37. Jahr JS, Lurie F, Gosselin R, et al. Effects of a hemoglobin-based oxygen carrier (HBOC-201) on coagulation testing. Clin Lab Sci 2000;13:210–4.

38. Shirey RS, Lewin M, Ness PM, et al. Hemoglobin-based oxygen carriers: effect on serologic pretransfusion testing. Transfusion 2004;44:122A.

39. Wolthuis A, Peek D, Scholten R, et al. Effect of the hemoglobin-based oxygen carrier HBOC-201 on laboratory instrumentation: cobas integra, chiron blood gas analyzer 840, Sysmex SE-9000 and BCT. Clin Chem Lab Med 1999;37: 71–6.

40. Kazmierczak SC, Catrou PG, Best AE, et al. Multiple regression analysis of inter-ference effects from a hemoglobin-based oxygen carrier solution. Clin Chem Lab Med 1999;37:453–64.

41. Callas DD, Clark TL, Moreira PL, et al. In vitro effects of a novel hemoglobin-based oxygen carrier on routine chemistry, therapeutic drug, coagulation, hema-tology, and blood bank assays. Clin Chem 1997;43:1744–8.

42. Jahr JS, Osgood S, Rothenberg SJ, et al. Lactate measurement interference by hemoglobin-based oxygen carriers (Oxyglobin, Hemopure, and Hemolink). Anesth Analg 2005;100:431–6.

43. Sakai H, Tomiyama K, Masada Y, et al. Pretreatment of serum containing hemo-globin vesicles (oxygen carriers) to prevent their interference in laboratory tests. Clin Chem Lab Med 2003;41:222–31.

44. Mullon J, Giacoppe G, Clagett C, et al. Transfusions of polymerized bovine hemoglobin in a patient with severe autoimmune hemolytic anemia. N Engl J Med 2000;342:1638–43.
45. Natanson C, Kern SJ, Lurie P, et al. Cell-free hemoglobin-based blood substitutes and risk of myocardial infarction and death: a meta-analysis. JAMA 2008;299: 2304–12.
46. Fergusson DA, McIntyre L. The future of clinical trials evaluating blood substitutes. JAMA 2008;299:2324–6.

The Ideal Blood Substitute

A. Gerson Greenburg, MD, PhD[a,b]

KEYWORDS

- Blood • Blood substitute • Hemoglobin
- Homeostasis • Transfusion

In writing this article, I take the prerogative of a senior investigator in the field of blood substitutes to express my opinions and views of what constitutes an ideal blood substitute. My perspective, based on a 35-year involvement with wide-ranging contributions from chemical modification of hemoglobin (Hb) to improve its characteristics as a "blood substitute" through the design and evaluation of Phase III clinical trials is perhaps unique in that regard. I have no doubt that there is a need for a blood substitute now and in the near future. In this article, I address some of the key elements to consider, offer some guidelines, and place a context on my suggestions in light of known physiology.

BLOOD

Blood is indisputably essential for life, and specifying the attributes of a solution to replace the life force of blood is a daunting task. An appreciation of the composition and structure of blood in the context of its many functions is an essential prerequisite for listing design specifications of an ideal blood substitute (IBS). Only by understanding the functions of blood is it possible to define the characteristics needed for an IBS.

The chief functions of blood are the provision of tissue perfusion with oxygen carried by the red cells' Hb and maintenance of vascular volume. Loss of vascular volume, as in trauma or operative surgery with loss of red cell mass, has widely known undesirable clinical consequences. In addition, blood provides cellular and molecular elements of the coagulation and immune systems and, by providing the vascular volume, serves as a communication pathway for hormonal and cytokine signaling and the delivery of nutrients and removal of metabolic waste products. Within each of these broader categories there are subsets of elements and components with complex interactions and functions that serve to maintain life and homeostasis, and participate in the protective responses to injury and the restorative processes required. Within each functional component there is an optimal operating level and

[a] Biopure Corporation, 11 Hurley Street, Cambridge, MA 02141, USA
[b] Brown University, Providence, RI, USA
E-mail address: aggreenburgmdphd@gmail.com

Crit Care Clin 25 (2009) 415–424
doi:10.1016/j.ccc.2009.01.004
0749-0704/09/$ – see front matter © 2009 Elsevier Inc. All rights reserved.

reserve capacity to respond to acute needs. An IBS would, de facto, have to replace all of these functions.

Given the prominence of the need to perfuse tissue with oxygen, the role of Hb and intravascular volume replacement has consumed and attracted great attention in the pursuit of an IBS. Replacing the lost oxygen-carrying capacity of blood, whether from hemorrhage or disease, has been an objective of much research. Failing to replace lost oxygen-carrying capacity, Hb perpetrates impaired tissue perfusion with consequent critical organ ischemic injury, initiating a downward spiral of organ failure, multi-system organ failure, and death. The need to avoid this sequence of events has driven the development of blood substitutes for over a century.

In the past 25 years, concerns about the safety of the blood supply and the inventory of available red cells as well as issues with storage, the quality of stored red blood cells and their impact on function and immune consequences and the potential for transmission of infectious disease have encouraged further development. Currently, an alternative to red blood cells as treatment does not exist. In the event of a major disaster or epidemic there is no available replacement. Stockpiles of red blood cells beyond the normal storage cycle of days do not exist. The availability of an option, even one that addresses only some of blood's functions while relying on the reserve capacity of the system for some of the other functions, is certainly a desirable goal. Indeed, faced with the nonavailability of blood for whatever reasons, restoring the oxygen-carrying capacity to the cardiovascular system until red cells are available is a reasonable bridge to definitive treatment.

An oxygen-carrying IBS to treat hemorrhagic shock or symptomatic acute blood loss as observed from time to time in surgical settings across all surgical specialties is preferable to standard asanguinous fluid therapy. The treatment of anemia and its consequences of ischemic insult for patients with primary hematologic malignancy or the side effect of chemotherapy could be enhanced, thus permitting patients to receive treatment otherwise denied, particularly if they object to blood transfusion. When blood is not available or otherwise not an option, the therapeutic armamentarium would be significantly enhanced with the inclusion of an IBS.

FORMULATION

Is there really an ideal blood substitute, a multipurpose formulation that would mimic the full functionality of blood or, as might be reasoned from the potential range of applications, could be formulated into separate solutions for separate applications? Should the properties be maximized for directed application or optimized for general use? The decision taken at this point has significant implications for the eventual formulation, for it will define the characteristics of the proposed solution. Matching form to function is a critical design element.

In the case of new therapeutic products, one needs an appreciation of the underlying mechanisms of disease and the influence they might have on the safety and effectiveness of any new approach. Understanding the pathophysiology to be treated is essential for the design and formulation of an IBS for that disease. It also permits differentiation of disease effects from treatment-associated effects during the critical safety analysis.

In my opinion, the "ideal blood substitute" is fresh whole blood, an autologous donation achieved by intraoperative hemodilution. With all the cellular and molecular components and functionality necessary and none of the safety issues associated with passage through the blood bank, it meets all the needs all the time. Unfortunately, this solution is not applicable to all situations, leaving the question of the specifications for an IBS of clinical use.

Although there are efforts to develop replacements for white cell function, coagulation, and immune functions in addition to the red cells' oxygen-carrying capacity, it is the latter that has captured the imagination of investigators over the past quarter century. The replacement of oxygen-carrying capacity has driven the field, primarily with the development of hemoglobin-based oxygen carriers (HBOCs), which for the moment comprise existing blood substitutes. At the current stage of development, the form of an IBS must have the ability to carry and deliver oxygen to tissues, maintaining and restoring organ perfusion and, ideally, homeostasis. The remainder of this commentary deals with HBOCs, as they have the longest history with respect to the development of an IBS.

CHARACTERISTICS

Any innovative treatment requires demonstration of an acceptable safety profile, relative to the intended indication. Safety is most often cast as a benefit/risk analysis. Whereas HBOCs are intended to replace hemorrhagic blood loss, avoiding death, the outcome logically would demand a different benefit/risk ratio from that necessary for avoidance of a red blood cell (RBC) transfusion. Extrapolating clinically defined safety data from elective surgical trials whereby the HBOC is pitted against packed RBC transfusion to other clinical situations requires some modulation of the safety standards. The evaluation of safety is a complex process, not well standardized, and complicated by the differing endpoints of trials and protocols for evaluation relative to proposed indications. Important is the recognition of the close relationship of safety and efficacy in evaluating an HBOC.

Efficacy is defined in terms of achieving the HBOC's objective, linked to the indication and thus related to the safety evaluation. Saving a life is not directly comparable to avoiding an RBC transfusion. Achieving endpoints within an acceptable safety profile appropriate to the indication and patient population is critical. Often, to understand some trial-emerging safety signals it is necessary to delve beyond the intent-to-treat analysis, a "gold standard," and apply clinical contextualization to provide an alternative explanation for the adverse event or events in question.

OXYGEN DELIVERY

As a substitute for the oxygen-carrying capacity of blood, a primary function of the RBC, the HBOC must demonstrate the ability to carry and deliver oxygen to tissues. Thus it follows that the Hb concentration of the HBOC ([Hb]) must be sufficient to meet the needs of the indication. Global oxygen delivery is governed by cardiac output and [Hb]. To increase oxygen delivery both need to be considered. It is easier to increase the amount of Hb, the oxygen-carrying capacity, than to risk driving cardiac output up, especially in the elderly or patients with cardiac disease. In most situations the indication is most likely the treatment of blood loss anemia and a solution with [Hb] equal to that of whole blood is reasonable. Indeed, for general use, a [Hb] of 12–15 gm/dL is sufficient. There may be situations whereby a greater or more rapid increase in tissue perfusion is desirable, eg, prolonged hypoperfusion or accumulated oxygen debt. In those cases, an HBOC with greater [Hb], say 20–25 gm/dL, could be useful. Creating a solution with this [Hb] is a significant challenge in formulation and process chemistry that needs to be addressed. If this level of [Hb] is deemed necessary for an ideal solution, then the problem must be resolved. From an efficacy standpoint, competition with packed RBCs with a higher concentration of Hb is difficult.

Competition with whole blood, were it available, would be reasonable, whereas competition with crystalloid and colloid solutions is clearly favorable to the solution that carries oxygen.

Oxy–hemoglobin affinity, expressed as P_{50} (the partial pressure of oxygen at which Hb is half-saturated) is another factor in the totality of oxygen delivery physiology to be considered. Removing Hb from its protective RBC membrane results in a significant decrease in P_{50} for the residual "stroma-free" native Hb. An increased oxy–Hb affinity of greater than 50% could play a role in altering oxygen delivery physiology dynamics. Historically, in the development of HBOCs, this was recognized and became one of the key drivers behind efforts to chemically modify Hb, eliminating this as a variable of concern.

Optimized to "normal" has been an objective for most HBOCs and some solutions have exceeded the 26–28 mm Hg P_{50} of intracellular Hb by as much as 50%. Acellular bovine Hb has a higher P_{50} than intracellular human Hb and its affinity is regulated by chloride ion and not 2,3–diphosphoglycerate present in the red cell of humans. A P_{50} for an HBOC from 30 to 45 mm Hg under standard conditions would be reasonable. Solutions with significantly lower P_{50} have been formulated and tested based on extrapolation from microcirculatory studies in animals. These lower P_{50} solutions and the affinity of myoglobin may serve more as intravascular oxygen storage than participating in direct offloading of oxygen to tissues for metabolic activity. It must be recognized that P_{50} is one element of oxygen delivery that is generally poorly appreciated.

Perhaps not as crucial a factor as [Hb] or cardiac output, the product of those two factors driving global oxygen delivery, the affinity of oxygen for Hb does play a role in oxygen delivery and use. With affinity increases, Hb binds oxygen more tightly (decreased P_{50}) and tissues are at risk of being deprived of oxygen, a functional deficit in oxygen delivery. With decreased affinity oxygen offloads more easily in the tissues. There is then the potential for an overabundance of oxygen locally in an area of previous ischemia, with the possibility of generating reactive oxygen species that could be harmful. These effects have not been demonstrated in clinical situations with HBOC. It is considered a hypothesis in search of evidence to demonstrate they do appear and are related, causally, to the appearance of adverse events. Under normal circumstances, the P_{50} is likely a minor factor in overall oxygen delivery physiology. Under conditions of stress, anaerobic metabolism, and increased oxygen demand by tissues, it could be a critical factor and the HBOC or IBS should have a P_{50} closer to the range noted above.

A NOTE ON CHEMISTRY

The additional chemistry to achieve this [Hb] likely involves additional modification of Hb and the possibility of the appearance of new or previously unrecognized safety signals. In achieving the desired functionality new issues may arise.

Chemical modification of Hb to achieve some or all of the desirable properties, attributes, and optimized levels of specific parameters will have a variety of forms. Included are tetrameric stabilization, conjugation with other molecules (eg, starches), polymerization, and encapsulation. Each modification approach has its own unique and intrinsic set of properties that add a dimension and presumed value to the product produced by the specific modification. Independent of the modification approach used, the general properties of the IBS or HBOC must be met. Additions to the solution to enhance physiologic function or storage parameters are part of the design process. A complete understanding of the contribution of each element is necessary to appreciate the impact on safety concerns. There is a potential for problematic additive or synergistic effects.

An ideal IBS or HBOC must act as a bridge in providing tissue perfusion until the patient recovers their own red cell mass or blood becomes available if needed.

HALF-LIFE

Circulating plasma half-life and oxygen affinity are other elements to consider. The ideal or desired half-life depends on the intended indication; function follows need. As a replacement for lost blood volume, hemorrhagic shock, plasma persistence until the availability of definitive red cell therapy would be appropriate. Unfortunately this is not always a known duration. The liquid acellular nature of HBOCs guarantees a significantly shorter plasma persistence than red blood cells, hours compared with days; persistence for days has not been achieved. For applications directed at ischemic rescue, for example, myocardial infarction, stroke, or acute peripheral limb arterial occlusion, a shorter circulating half-life is not unreasonable. In general, an optimized circulating half-life of 18–24 hours would suffice for most currently projected applications.

VISCOSITY

Fluid viscosity is a property that affects vascular tone and thus vasoactivity. The viscosity of the clinically tested HBOCs ranges from considerably less than that of plasma and blood to levels considerably higher. The issue with claiming that viscosity has an impact on adverse events and vasoactivity in particular is the inability to identify a direct correlation between observed events. It is difficult to differentiate the impact and effect of viscosity on vasoactivity from other components of the solution clinically or in the models used to explore the effect, thus it is not clear what the viscosity should be. Like oxy–hemoglobin affinity, P_{50}, viscosity may play a role in the overall physiologic response to HBOC infusions. Although the ideal viscosity for an HBOC has not been identified, a value near to plasma would be acceptable.

VASOACTIVITY

Vasoactivity has been implicated in some of the adverse events noted with infusion of HBOC solutions. An ideal HBOC or IBS would of necessity address this issue and demonstrate that it is (a) a "side-effect" of the drug, treatable and without lasting consequence, (b) a beneficial effect in some clinical situations, or (c) truly the causative agent of serious adverse events and toxicity. A commonly held concept and working hypothesis used to explain the emergence of serious adverse events associated with the use of the current HBOCs is vasoactivity and an elevation of blood pressure. While some elevation in blood pressure, an increased perfusion pressure, may be appropriate for some indications, for example, stroke and traumatic brain injury, the observation of an unpredictable significant increase in blood pressure in some trials has raised this question to great visibility. The blood pressure response, generally about 15–25 mm Hg systolic, seems to be associated with the concentration of tetrameric Hb present in the formulation; a greater increase in blood pressure is observed in those formulations with more tetramer. To counter this long-recognized effect, chemical modification of Hb to minimize tetrameric Hb in the solution has been used with some success. While minimizing the amount of tetramer there is a gain in prolonging the intravascular persistence, a desirable characteristic.

It is a widely and generally held notion that elimination of the vasoactivity of an HBOC or IBS will reduce the so-called "toxicity" as expressed in the incidence of serious cardiac, cerebral and renal adverse events. It is not clear that vasoactivity to the point of true hypertension always happens or that the clinical scenarios where it is more likely to be seen have been identified. From the clinical perspective it appears to be unpredictable as to incidence and degree. The mechanism is ascribed to Hb in the HBOC-scavenging nitric oxide (NO), a major participant in the regulation of vascular tone as a vasodilator. Significant efforts to design newer HBOCs directed at resolving this issue have achieved some success. Additional polymerization, the use of additives to induce vasodilation, replacing the consumed NO with nitrate and nitrite compounds have all been proposed but not yet clinically tested. One point is clear, however: if decreased vasoactivity is achieved at the expense of decreasing [Hb], a decrease in oxygen-carrying capacity of the HBOC, the resultant solution will be compromised with respect to increasing global oxygen delivery and tissue perfusion.

In my clinical experience in treating patients with an HBOC, elevations in blood pressure have been observed. In instances where a concern about the magnitude of the increase was expressed, routine clinical interventions (eg, beta blockers, nitrate donors, or calcium channel blockers) have modulated the effect safely and the patients experienced no long-term sequelae. In my clinical opinion and based on hard analysis of Phase III trial data there is no firm clinical data to relate vasoactivity to the "toxicity" of HBOCs.

Absent proof of a direct relationship of vasoactivity and serious adverse events in an acceptable logically described causal argument, an ideal HBOC can have the property of vasoactivity with increases of 25% in blood pressure over the baseline pressure at the start of the infusion. Given that many of the indications are for situations where there is acute blood loss and hypotension, this is not an unreasonable increase that can be modulated if necessary.

Chemical modification stabilizes the Hb molecule and, by enlarging it into polymers with a range of size distributions, decreases the rate of clearance from the circulation. In addition, the increase in molecular size decreases the number of protein particles and helps to produce a solution with an acceptable oncotic pressure. This is another property of concern in the overall design of an ideal HBOC or IBS. Despite the wide range over which an oncotic pressure can vary without inducing significant shifts in fluid compartments, maintaining this parameter near normal for an ideal formulation is reasonable.

STORAGE AND STABILITY

A long shelf life and temperature stable storage are other desirable properties. The concept of stockpiling a red cell substitute for disasters is very appealing. Storage for three years at room temperature is offered as one standard, extendable with freezing or refrigeration. However, for clinical use, especially in trauma situations with long transport times, refrigeration might be an issue. Refrigerated transport in emergency vehicles or for use out of hospital cannot always be accommodated. The product deliverable after storage, independent of modality, must meet all of the functional, chemical, and stability characteristics of the original product with respect to all of its characteristics including [Hb], P_{50}, molecular weight distribution, oncotic pressure, osmolality, and oxidative state. Each of these parameters has a manufacturing specification and storage should not induce any significant variation over the time afforded by the label. The protein cannot precipitate nor oxidize to methemoglobin (metHb) in storage. The solution should be ready to use directly from the sterile endotoxin-free storage container without the need to mix additives or thaw or warm the product, steps that would complicate and possibly compromise use.

EXCIPIENT

The excipient, the carrier solvent for the Hb, is another variable of concern raised by some investigators. A balanced salt solution, Ringer's Lactate or Ringer's Acetate, modulates the osmolality and has been generally used in the formulations. There are some who feel that the D–lactate fraction of the mixed L–D Ringer's solution may play a role in the emergence of some of the observed adverse events, especially in patients with diabetes. A balanced salt solution excipient minimizes infusion of free water and provides electrolytes to maintain osmotic pressure. As there have been little or no data forthcoming, beyond intellectual property rights to support an advantage of any one cation over another, there is none to be specified for the ideal HBOC.

STERILITY AND IMMUNOLOGY

The ideal HBOC is endotoxin-free and the source material of Hb is certifiably disease-free as well. Monitoring for the introduction of pathogens or the presence of endotoxin during the manufacturing at all steps is required. The ideal HBOC meets all the necessary certifications for manufacture of a parenteral pharmaceutical as well as GMP specifications. The source of the Hb molecule must be traceable. In the case of animal sources, bovine, porcine, or ovine, the absence of animal-carried pathogens and vectors must be assured. If the Hb is produced by recombinant technology, all evidence of the vectors and production methodology must be removed.

Chemical modification creates a modified protein, a new epitope of Hb, raising concern about the immunogenicity of the resultant product. From clinical experience, when first infused or infused over a number of days, no severe immune responses have been observed. If the Hb is of nonhuman source there is the possibility of a reaction from prior exposure, and careful labeling of the product and questioning of the patients should elicit the information needed to withhold the indicated infusion if necessary. Given the chemical modification of the Hb, some degree of immunogenicity is expected, although not fully appreciated with concerns expressed regarding issues with delayed expression or responses to subsequent exposures. The ideal HBOC does not induce an immune response upon infusion nor does it compromise the immune system function, especially in trauma patients or those with pre-existing immune compromise. Minimal impact on the immune system is a very desirable characteristic.

In the early years of HBOC development there were concerns about nephrotoxicity and coagulopathy. They persist today despite overwhelming clinical evidence that these adverse events, so-called "toxicities," are not really issues. There is still a low incidence of compromised renal function associated with the use of HBOCs that, on closer examination, seems to be the result of underlying pre-existing renal disease or inadequate treatment of hypovolemia. The current manufacturing and production methods for HBOCs are very efficient at eliminating the red cell stroma which has been shown to be the primary source of the product-related renal problems and coagulopathy observed in the past. An ideal HBOC has no detectable lipoprotein concentrations, red cell membrane fragments; their removal is essential to producing a useful infusate. Of course, establishing the chemical purity of each component of the solution, active or inert, is also essential. That includes additives that assist in storage stabilization.

CLEARANCE AND METABOLISM

The ideal HBOC has minimal impact on the cytokine cascade, an integral part of the immune and coagulation systems. In situations where an HBOC is likely to be used, for example, trauma, acute blood loss, chemotherapy, or blood is not an option, these critical homeostatic systems/mechanisms are already perturbed, and any additional stress could uncouple the entire homeostatic response mechanism. A therapeutic agent that further compromises an essential physiologic system is not desirable and suppressing the immune system, lowering the host defense mechanisms, is also an undesirable characteristic. Thus, the ideal HBOC should not impair the function of the reticuloendothelial system (RES) or the other components of the host defense mechanism. Current HBOCs are thought to be cleared by the RES and some of these mechanisms may well be protective, metabolizing the product via pathways that are anti-inflammatory and thus protective against some of the metabolic pro-inflammatory responses perhaps responsible for some of the adverse events. The ideal HBOC should not impair or have a lasting impact on the host defense mechanisms or coagulation systems. The absence of teratogenicity is of course a requirement.

The Hb added must be metabolized. This is generally facilitated in the RES as noted. In clinical experience the exposed iron of the heme-groups on the Hb are subject to oxidation, the formation of met-Hb. When present it decreases the functional delivery of oxygen, not dissimilar to the effect of P_{50} changes, as there are few reducing substances in the plasma. While it is preferable to eliminate the formation of met-Hb this may not be possible. Thus, approaches to minimize its impact, such as providing reducing agents during the therapy, prophylactically or therapeutically, may be necessary.

LABORATORY ISSUES

The ideal HBOC has no interference issues with laboratory testing. However, as many of the modern laboratory techniques employ optical methodology this may be an unattainable goal. A complete manual of test interference for the ideal HBOC is a requirement.

SUMMARY

The ideal blood substitute meets the needs of the situation or disease for which it is being used, primarily as a bridge until red cells are available or when blood is not an option or is not available. The formulation is optimized to provide tissue perfusion for maintenance and restoration of function and preserve organ integrity. And it is composed in such a way as to minimize additional organ compromise or interfere with homeostatic and compensatory physiologic mechanisms. It has an acceptable safety profile and certainly is not toxic. Universal compatibility is expected and use without typing or cross-matching is required. While it has "side-effects" that are transient and treatable, it has no intrinsic toxicity to vital organs. It is shelf storable, ready to use, complete in its formulation to achieve the objective. It is producible at reasonable cost. There is an ongoing need for a red cell substitute, an oxygen-carrying solution for use in many clinical situations. A complete substitute for blood with all the cellular and molecular components of the immune and coagulation systems is a distant dream. For now, efforts must be focused on developing effective and safe oxygen therapeutics.

APPENDIX

A list of selected readings is provided to permit the reader access to some of the thinking behind the development of HBOCs over the past 60 years. It is not an all-inclusive reference set. Rather, for the interested reader, it provides a starting point for exploring the history of the concepts behind the development of these potentially useful solutions addressing the issues relevant to the design of an ideal blood substitute.

FURTHER READINGS

Amberson WR, Jennings JJ, Rhode CM. Clinical experience with hemoglobin–saline solutions. J Appl Physiol 1949;1(7):469–89.

Carmichael FJL, Ali ACY, Campbell J, et al. A phase I study of oxidized raffinose cross-linked human hemoglobin. Crit Care Med 2000;vol 28(7):2283–92.

Chang TM. Future generations of red blood cell substitutes. J Intern Med 2003;253: 527–35.

Chang TM. Opening keynote lecture (OKL). 50th anniversary of artificial cells: evolving to oxygen carriers, oxygen therapeutics, nano artificial RBC and a novel oxygen carrier with platelet-like function. Artif Cells Blood Substit Immobil Biotechnol 2008;36(3):181–4.

Cutcliffe NE, Carmichael FJ, Greenburg AG. Blood substitutes: a review of clinical trials. In: Mathiowitz E, editor. The encyclopedia of controlled drug delivery. New York: John Wiley & Sons, Inc.; 1999. p. 94–112.

Dube GP, Vranckx P, Greenburg AG. HBOC-201: the multipurpose oxygen therapeutic. EuroIntervention 2008;4:161–5.

Estep T, Bucci E, Farmer M, et al. Basic science focus on blood substitutes: a summary of the NHLBI Division of Blood Diseases and Resources Working Group Workshop, March 1, 2006. Transfusion 2008;48:776–82.

Greenburg AG, Pearl J, Belsha J, et al. An improved stroma-free hemoglobin solution. Surg Forum 1975;26:53–5.

Greenburg AG, Hayshi R, Krupenas I, et al. Intravascular persistence and oxygen delivery of pyridoxalated stroma-free hemoglobin during gradations of hypotension. Surgery 1979;86:13–6.

Greenburg AG, Peskin GW, Hoyt DB, et al. Is it necessary to improve the intravascular retention of hemoglobin solutions. Crit Care Med 1982;10:266–9.

Greenburg AG. The effects of hemoglobin on reticuloendothelial function. In: Bolin RB, Geyer RP, Nemo GJ, editors. Advances in Blood Substitute Research. New York: Alan R. Liss, Inc.; 1983. p. 127–37.

Greenburg AG, Kim HW, The Hemolink Study Group. The use of an oxygen therapeutic as an adjunct to intraoperative autologous donation to reduce transfusion requirements in patients undergoing coronary artery bypass surgery. J Am Coll Surg 2004;vol 198(No. 3):373–85.

Greenburg AG, Pitman A, Pearce LB, et al. Clinical contextualization and the assessment of adverse events in HBOC trials. Artif Cells Blood Substit Immobil Biotechnol 2008;36:477–86.

Jahr JS, Mackenzie C, Pearce LB, et al. HBOC-201 as an alternative to blood transfusion: efficacy and safety evaluation in a multicenter phase III trial in elective orthopedic surgery. J Trauma 2008;64:1484–97.

Kim HW, Awad M, Greenburg AG. Coagulation responses of human plasma after hemodilution with hemoglobin solution in vitro. Artif Cells Blood Substit Immobil Biotechnol 1994;22(3):613–8.

Kim HW, Greenburg AG. Hemoglobin-mediated vasoactivity in isolated vascular rings. Artif Cells Blood Substit Immobil Biotechnol 1995;23:303–10.

Kim HW, Greenburg AG. Engineered hemoglobins as potential therapeutics: from red cell substitutes to cancer therapy adjuvants, Proceedings of the 1996 Korean Federation of Scientists and Engineers International Technical Conference (6/24-28/96, Korea); 1996. p. 1300–7.

Kim HW, Greenburg AG. Mechanisms for vasoconstriction and decreased blood flow following intravenous administration of cell-free native hemoglobin solutions. Adv Exp Med Biol 2005;566:397–401.

Kim HW, Greenburg AG. Artificial oxygen carriers as red blood cell substitutes: a selected review and current status. Artif Organs 2004;28:819–28.

Natanson C, Kern SJ, Lurie P, et al. Cell-free hemoglobin-based blood substitutes and risk of myocardial infarction and death: a meta-analysis. JAMA 2008;299(19): 2304–12. A commentary on this analysis is. Available at: http://www.biopure.com. Accessed September 1, 2008.

Natanson C. Incomplete financial disclosure in a study of cell-free hemoglobin-based blood substitutes and risks of myocardial infarction and death. JAMA 2008;300(11): 1300 (relates to previous citation).

Ness PM, Cushing MM. Oxygen therapeutics: pursuit of an alternative to the donor red cell. Arch Pathol Lab Med 2007;131:734–41.

Ravdin IS, Fitts WT Jr. The so-called "blood substitutes". Am J Surg 1950;80:744–52.

Savitsky JP, Doczi J, Black J, et al. A clinical safety trial of stroma-free hemoglobin. Clin Pharmacol Ther 1978;23:73–80.

Whitley D, Patterson R, Greenburg AG. Cell-free hemoglobin preserves renal function during normothermic ischemia. J Surg Res 1998;77:187–91.

Winslow RM. Historical background in blood substitutes. In: Winslow RM, editor. Elsevier Inc.; 2006. p. 5–16, Chapter 1.

Index

Note: Page numbers of article titles are in **boldface** type.

A

Anemia(s)
    physiology of, 262–264
    sickle cell, HBOCs for, 318
Arterial blood, oxygen content of, calculation of, 263

B

Baxter Hemoglobin Therapeutics, 283
Biodegradable polymeric nanodimension artificial RBCs, 378–380
Blood
    arterial, oxygen content of, calculation of, 263
    described, 415–416
    supply of, concerns related to, 416
Blood loss, perioperative, HBOCs for, 315–316
Blood substitutes
    functions of, 415–416
    gastrointestinal, 406–407
    HBOCs as, 314–316
    hematologic, 407
    hemoglobin-based, nanobiotechnology for, **373–382**
    ideal, 400, **415–424**
        characteristics of, 416–417
        chemistry of, 418–419
        clearance of, 422
        excipient, 421
        formulation of, 416–417
        half-life of, 419
    immunologic, 406
    immunology of, 421
    infectious, 407
    laboratory issues in, 422
    metabolism of, 422
    neurovascular, 405–406
    oxygen delivery and, 417–418
    safety of, 405–407
    stability of, 420–421
    sterility of, 421
    storage of, 420–421
    testing interference related to, 407–408
    toxicities of, 405–407

Crit Care Clin 25 (2009) 425–430
doi:10.1016/S0749-0704(09)00027-X
0749-0704/09/$ – see front matter © 2009 Elsevier Inc. All rights reserved.

criticalcare.theclinics.com

Blood (*continued*)
vasoactivity of, 419–420
viscosity of, 419
Blood transfusion
alternatives to, reasons for, **261–277**
contraindications to, 271–272
costs of, 270–271
outcomes of, 269
physiology of, 262–264
risks associated with, 265–270

C

CBER. See *Center for Biologics Evaluation and Research (CBER)*.
Cellular HBOCs, 294–295
Center for Biologics Evaluation and Research (CBER), 326
Critical care medicine, HBOCs in, potential uses, **311–324**

E

Embryo, as source of embryonic stem cells, 389–393
Endothelial permeability, hemoglobin-induced, 365

F

Fetus, as source of embryonic stem cells, 389–393
Fluid(s), transfusion, rHb for, design of, **357–371**. See also *Recombinant hemoglobin (rHb), in transfusion fluids*.

H

HBOCs. See *Hemoglobin-based oxygen carriers (HBOCs)*.
Heart, tetrameric hemoglobin in polyhemoglobin effects on, 374–375
Hematopoiesis, 384–385
Heme-pocket mutations, 359–362
Hemoglobin
as red blood cell substitute, 280
polymerized, in trauma care. See *Polymerized hemoglobin, in trauma care*.
structure of, 280
tetrameric, modified, in trauma care, clinical evaluation of, 327–328
Hemoglobin polymerization, 363–365
"Hemoglobin therapeutic," HBOCs as, 317–318
Hemoglobin-based blood substitutes, nanobiotechnology for, **373–382**. See also *Nanobiotechnology, for hemoglobin-based blood substitutes*.
Hemoglobin-based oxygen carriers (HBOCs), **279–301,** 284
adverse effects of, 296–297
as blood substitute, 314–316
as "hemoglobin therapeutic," 317–318
cellular, 294–295
characteristics of, 304–306
comparison to stored packed RBCs, **303–310**
described, 307–308
described, 279–283

first-generation, 283
for myocardial infarction, 318
for sepsis, 317–318
for septic shock, 317–318
for sickle cell anemia, 318
for stroke, 318
formation of, 280
gastrointestinal side effects of, 296
hemostasis of, 296
in hemorrhagic shock, 314–315
in perioperative blood losses, 315–316
in trauma care, 314–315
    potential clinical benefits of, 326
    potential role of, 325–327
interference with laboratory assays, 296
next generation, 293–295
oncotic effects of, 312–313
oxygen-carrying capacity of, 312
potential uses in critical care medicine, **311–324**
    described, 311–312
problems related to, 281–282
products in clinical trials, 283–293
    HemoLink, 289–291
    Hemopure, 284–287
    MP4, 291–293
    PolyHeme, 284, 288–289
properties of, 312–314
vasoactivity of, 296
vasopressor effects of, 313–314
Hemoglobin-based oxygen carriers (HBOCs) interference, 408–410
Hemoglobin-induced endothelial permeability, 365
HemoLink, 289
clinical trials of, 289–291
Hemopure, 284
clinical trials of, 284–287
Hemorrhagic shock
acute, polymerized hemoglobin for, 333–334
HBOCs in, 314–315

M

Maleimide PEG-Hb (MP4), 291
clinical trials of, 291–293
Modified tetrameric hemoglobin, in trauma care, clinical evaluation of, 327–328
MP4 (Maleimide PEG-Hb), 291
clinical trials of, 291–293
Mutation(s)
Heme-pocket, 359–362
surface, 362
Myocardial infarction, HBOCs for, 318
Myoglobin, as oxygen transporter and plasma expander, 367

N

Nanobiotechnology, **373–382**
   described, 373
   directions in, 380
   for hemoglobin-based blood substitutes, **373–382**
      assembling hemoglobin with catalase and superoxide dismutase, 375–377
      biodegradable polymeric nanodimension artificial RBCs, 378–380
      new generation of, 375–377
National Heart, Lung, and Blood Institute, 282

O

Oxygen content of arterial blood, calculation of, 263
Oxygen delivery
   blood substitutes and, 417–418
   rHb and, 365–367
Oxygen therapeutics, **399–414**
   described, 399–400
Oxygen transport, physiology of, 262–264
Oxygen transporter, myoglobin as, 367
Oxygen-carrying capacity, of HBOCs, 312

P

Perfluorocarbons
   blood substitute safety and, **399–414**
   first commercial application of, 402
   history of, 401–404
   mechanism of action of, 401–404
   outlook for, 403
   second-generation, 402–403
Perfluorocarbons interference, 408
Plasma expander, myoglobin as, 367
PolyHeme, 288
   characteristics of, 304–305
   clinical trials of, 284, 288–289
Polyhemoglobin, 373–375
   basic principles of, 373–374
   in clinical trials, status of, 374
   tetrameric hemoglobin in
      cardiac effects of, 374–375
      vasoconstriction effects of, 374–375
Polyhemoglobin-fibrinogen, 377–378
   in vitro experiments, 377
   in vivo experiments, 378
Polymerization, hemoglobin, 363–365
Polymerized hemoglobin, in trauma care
   clinical efficacy of, 329–334
   clinical safety of, 328–329
   for acute hemorrhagic shock, 333–334
   perioperative applications of, 329–333

R

RBCs. See *Red blood cells (RBCs)*.
Recombinant hemoglobin (rHb), 293
    described, 358–359
    in transfusion fluids
        design of, **357–371**
        Heme-pocket mutations, 359–362
        hemoglobin polymerization, 363–365
        hemoglobin-induced endothelial permeability, 365
        need for, 357–358
        surface mutations, 362
    oxygen delivery and, 365–367
Red blood cells (RBCs)
    adult, for transfusion, stem cells for, **383–398.** See also *Stem cells, for transfusion*.
    biodegradable polymeric nanodimension artificial, 378–380
    production of, in laboratory, objectives for, 385–389
    replacement of
        described, 383–384
        hematopoiesis, 384–385
        perspectives on, 389
        possibility of, 383–389
        prerequisites for, 385
    stored packed
        characteristics of, 306–307
        comparison to HBOCs, **303–310**
rHb. See *Recombinant hemoglobin (rHb)*.

S

Sepsis, HBOCs for, 317–318
Septic shock, HBOCs for, 317–318
Shock
    hemorrhagic
        acute, polymerized hemoglobin for, 333–334
        HBOCs in, 314–315
    septic, HBOCs for, 317–318
Sickle cell anemia, HBOCs for, 318
Stem cells
    for transfusion, **383–398**
        adult pluripotent sources of, 393–396
        fetal and embryonic sources of, 389–393
    multipotent
        adult progenitor cells as, 393
        diverse potential sources of, 394
    patient-specific, 394
    pluripotent, induced, 394–396
    unrestricted somatic, 393–394
Stroke, HBOCs for, 318
Surface mutations, 362

T

Tetrameric hemoglobin, modified, in trauma care, clinical evaluation of, 327–328
Transfusion(s)
    blood, alternative to, reasons for, **261–277.** See also *Blood transfusion.*
    physiology of, 262–264
    RBCs for, stem cells as source of, **383–398.** See also *Stem cells, for transfusion.*
Transfusion fluids, rHb for, design of, **357–371.** See also *Recombinant hemoglobin (rHb), in transfusion fluids.*
Trauma care
    HBOCs in, 314–315
        modified tetrameric hemoglobin in, clinical evaluation of, 327–328
        potential clinical benefits of, 326
        potential role of, 325–327
    polymerized hemoglobin in. See *Polymerized hemoglobin, in trauma care.*

U

USA Multicenter Prehospital HBOC Resuscitation Trial, **334–351**
    clinical implications of, 347–351
    cohort analyses, 338
    described, 334–336
    primary efficacy end point, 338
    results of, 338
    safety analyses, 339–347
    secondary efficacy endpoints, 338–339
    statistical analysis, 337–338
    study design, 336
    study end points, 336

V

Vasoconstriction, tetrameric hemoglobin in polyhemoglobin effects on, 374–375

Moving?

Make sure your subscription moves with you!

To notify us of your new address, find your **Clinics Account Number** (located on your mailing label above your name), and contact customer service at:

E-mail: elspcs@elsevier.com

800-654-2452 (subscribers in the U.S. & Canada)
314-453-7041 (subscribers outside of the U.S. & Canada)

Fax number: 314-523-5170

Elsevier Periodicals Customer Service
11830 Westline Industrial Drive
St. Louis, MO 63146

*To ensure uninterrupted delivery of your subscription, please notify us at least 4 weeks in advance of move.

Printed and bound by CPI Group (UK) Ltd, Croydon, CR0 4YY

03/10/2024

01040443-0019